The Junior Doctor's Guide to Cardiology

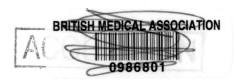

The Junior Doctor's Guide to Cardiology

IAN MANN
BMedSci (Hons), MBBS, MRCP
Core Medical Trainee Year 2
Royal Brompton Hospital

CHRISTOPHER CRITOPH
BM, MRCP
British Heart Foundation Research Fellow
The Heart Hospital
University College London

and

CAROLINE COATS
MBBS, BSc, MRCP, DHMSA
British Heart Foundation Research Fellow
The Heart Hospital
University College London

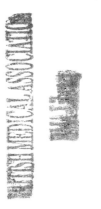

Foreword by
PETER COLLINS
Professor of Clinical Cardiology
National Heart and Lung Institute, Imperial College London
Honorary Consultant Cardiologist, Royal Brompton Hospital

Radcliffe Publishing
London • New York

Radcliffe Publishing Ltd
33–41 Dallington Street
London
EC1V 0BB
United Kingdom

www.radcliffepublishing.com

Electronic catalogue and worldwide online ordering facility.

British Library Cataloguing in Publication Data

A catalogue record for this book is available from the British Library.

ISBN-13: 978 184619 557 0

The paper used for the text pages of this book is FSC® certified. FSC (The Forest Stewardship Council®) is an international network to promote responsible management of the world's forests.

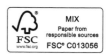

Typeset by Darkriver Design, Auckland, New Zealand
Printed and bound by TJI Digital, Padstow, Cornwall, UK

Contents

Foreword

It is a pleasure to write the Foreword to this excellent practical *The Junior Doctor's Guide to Cardiology*.

When I first entered medical school, a very wise senior tutor said to me, 'Collins, learn the basics and you won't go far wrong!' It has been a principle that has stayed with me throughout my medical career. The problem is in defining the basics and how to identify them. Information is becoming so freely available we risk being flooded and not all of the information is reliable. The trees, let alone the wood, can sometimes be very difficult to identify in this ever expanding specialty.

It is therefore so refreshing to see young physicians combining and producing a book for their (slightly!) younger colleagues with a genuine desire to help them through what is a confusing, difficult and sometimes lonely time. Trainees are often trying desperately to grapple with what appears to be massive amounts of new information in the very shortest time, often in a specialty in which they have had little exposure during their medical school career. As the authors point out, no sooner has a junior doctor started an attachment and settled in then it is time to move on again.

The European Working Time Directive has also shortened precious patient contact and clinical time, so much so that even when they are in training their exposure time is short. As well as providing excellent and up-to-date information this book deals with practical issues such as how to prioritise time and organise a ward round, which investigations to arrange and why. This may appear simple and straightforward information, but it can make an enormous difference to the day-to-day management of patients who are often in hospital for ever shorter periods of time. As cardiology is such a procedural specialty this information, acquired readily by a few nights' bedtime reading, will prove invaluable. It will also provide a welcome friend and ally whilst in the clinical arena.

I am sure this book will help you and hopefully entice you into the wonderful and expanding world of cardiology – good luck and don't forget 'learn the basics!'

Peter Collins
Professor of Clinical Cardiology
National Heart and Lung Institute, Imperial College London
Honorary Consultant Cardiologist, Royal Brompton Hospital
June 2011

Preface

The transition between medical student and junior doctor is both stressful and demanding. The learning curve is extremely steep, and even more so in the world of specialist medicine. Junior doctors are expected to move around to different areas every 4 to 6 months. Although this provides excellent exposure, just as they are starting to get comfortable with the job, they have to move on to a new specialty. Senior doctors expect a lot of their juniors, often forgetting how complex much of their chosen specialty is. As a result, junior doctors often feel out of their depth, and may be too embarrassed to tell their seniors when they don't understand something.

The majority of books currently available on this subject are packed full of information, but much of this is not aimed at junior doctors working on the front line. These books often list countless investigations and areas of management for specific medical conditions. However, they lack explanation of the results you should expect to obtain from these investigations, and their interpretation in the clinical context. We have written this book to act as a 'user's guide' for junior doctors for day-to-day clinical cardiology while they are out on the wards. It should provide a logical stepwise guide through the more common problems encountered in cardiology, and support the junior doctor with their clinical practice and decision making.

We have all been in the situation where, as a junior, we request an investigation not because we are looking for a highly specific answer, but because our consultant has asked us to request it. We believe that this book helps to explain the reasons why an investigation is requested, and provides a basic understanding of how to interpret the result. Furthermore, we have included chapters covering areas such as successful ward rounds and safe prescribing in cardiology, which should further offer support for you as a junior doctor.

This book is primarily aimed at FY1 and FY2 doctors, to serve as a means of quick reference on the ward. We hope that it provides you with some user-friendly support which you can use in your daily clinical practice, and that it makes life slightly more comfortable for both you and your patients. Good luck!

Ian Mann
Chris Critoph
Caroline Coats
June 2011

About the authors

Dr Ian Mann graduated from St Bartholomew's and the Royal London School of Medicine and Dentistry in 2007, with distinctions in Clinical Practice and Clinical Science. He also gained a first-class Biomedical Sciences degree with honours in Molecular Therapeutics during his intercalated year at medical school. He then went on to gain his MRCP in November 2010 while working on the intensive care unit at the Royal Brompton.

Dr Mann is at present working in Cardiology at the Royal Brompton Hospital in his second year of the Core Medical Training Programme, and is currently applying for specialist registrar training in cardiology. He has a particular interest in electrophysiology, as well as general cardiology. He is also interested in medical education, and dedicates a large amount of his time to the ward-based teaching of medical students and nursing staff.

Dr Chris Critoph graduated from Southampton Medical School in 2001. He completed his MRCP in 2004 following a medical rotation in Wessex, before working in intensive care at a teaching hospital in Sydney for one year. On returning to the UK he worked as a cardiology registrar on the North East Thames Training Programme. His sub-specialty interests are heart muscle disease and devices. He is currently a British Heart Foundation Research Fellow working towards a research MD in cardiomyopathy at the Heart Hospital, University College London.

Dr Critoph has written cardiology MRCP exam questions for Oxford University Press, and has contributed a chapter to the most recent edition of the *Oxford Handbook of Cardiology*. He is the author of several interactive cardiology modules in the Department of Health e-learning programme for medical trainees.

Dr Caroline Coats graduated from King's College London in 1999 with a first class BSc in Physiology, and, subsequently from Imperial College School of Medicine in 2002. She completed her general medical training in Edinburgh and worked as a Cardiology Registrar in New Zealand before returning to London as an academic trainee.

Dr Coats is currently a PhD student and British Heart Foundation Research Fellow at University College London. Her clinical interests are heart failure and echocardiography, and her research interests are exercise physiology and cardiac metabolism. She is regularly involved in teaching undergraduates, with a particular emphasis on integrating basic sciences into clinical training. She has also been awarded the Osler Medal for History of Medicine.

Original line art by Dr Tau Boga, Cardiologist, Hutt Hospital, New Zealand.

List of abbreviations

ABC	Airway, breathing, circulation
ABG	Arterial blood gas
ACEi	Angiotensin-converting-enzyme inhibitor
ACTH	Adrenocorticotropic hormone
A&E	Accident and Emergency
AF	Atrial fibrillation
ALP	Alkaline phosphatase
ALS	Advanced life support
ANA	Antinuclear antibody
ANCA	Antineutrophil cytoplasmic antibody
AP	Anterior–posterior
AR	Aortic regurgitation
A2RB	Angiotensin-2-receptor blocker
ARVC	Arrhythmogenic right ventricular cardiomyopathy
ASA	Acetylsalicylic acid (aspirin)
ASD	Atrial septal defect
AST	Aspartate aminotransferase
AVM	Arterio-venous malformation
AVNRT	Atrioventricular nodal re-entry tachycardia
AVRT	Atrioventricular re-entry tachycardia
BNP	Brain natriuretic peptide
BP	Blood pressure
CABG	Coronary artery by-pass graft
CAD	Coronary artery disease
CCF	Congestive cardiac failure
CCU	Coronary care unit

CK	Creatine kinase
CMR	Cardiac magnetic resonance (imaging)
COPD	Chronic obstructive pulmonary disease
CPAP	Continuous positive airway pressure
CPR	Cardiopulmonary resuscitation
CRP	C-reactive protein
CRT	Cardiac resynchronisation therapy
CRT-D	Cardiac resynchronisation therapy with a defibrillator device
CRT-P	Cardiac resynchronisation therapy with a pacing device
CS	Cardiogenic shock
CT	Computer tomography
CTPA	Computer tomography pulmonary angiogram
CV	Cardiovascular
CVP	Central venous pressure
Cx	Circumflex
CXR	Chest X-ray
DBP	Diastolic blood pressure
DCCV	Direct current cardioversion
DIG	Digitalis Investigation Group
DM	Diabetes mellitus
DVT	Deep vein thrombosis
EBV	Epstein–Barr virus
ECG	Electrocardiogram
EF	Ejection fraction
ENA	Extractable nuclear antigen
EP	Electrophysiology
EPO	Erythropoietin
ESD	End systolic diameter
ESR	Erythrocyte sedimentation rate
ETT	Exercise tolerance testing
FBC	Full blood count
FHx	Family history
GA	General anaesthetic
GBM	Glomerular basement membrane
GCS	Glasgow Coma Scale
GFR	Glomerular filtration rate
GGT	Gamma-glutamyl transferase
GI	Gastrointestinal
GP	General practitioner
GTN	Glyceryl trinitrate

GU	Genito-urinary
GUCH	Grown-up congenital heart disease
HCM	Hypertrophic cardiomyopathy
HDU	High-dependency unit
HIV	Human immunodeficiency virus
HTN	Hypertension
IABP	Intra-aortic balloon pump
ICD	Implantable cardioverter defibrillator
ICU	Intensive care unit
IE	Infective endocarditis
IHD	Ischaemic heart disease
INR	International normalised ratio
IV	Intravenous
IVDU	Intravenous drug user
JVP	Jugular venous pressure
LA	Left atrium
LAD	Left anterior descending *or* left axis deviation
LBBB	Left bundle branch block
LCx	Left circumflex
LDH	Lactate dehydrogenase
LDL	Low-density lipoprotein
LFT	Liver function tests
LMWH	Low-molecular-weight heparin
LOC	Loss of consciousness
LV	Left ventricle
LVEDD	Left ventricular end diastolic diameter
LVEF	Left ventricular ejection fraction
LVESD	Left ventricular end systolic diameter
LVH	Left ventricular hypertrophy
LVOT	Left ventricular outflow tract
MAU	Medical assessment unit
MC&S	Microscopy, culture and sensitivity
MI	Myocardial infarction
MPS	Myocardial perfusion scan
MR	Mitral regurgitation
MRA	Magnetic resonance angiography
MRI	Magnetic resonance imaging
MRSA	Methicillin-resistant *Staphylococcus aureus*
NICE	National Institute for Health and Clinical Excellence
NSAID	Non-steroidal anti-inflammatory drug

NSTEMI	Non-ST elevation myocardial infarction
NYHA	New York Heart Association
OCP	Oral contraceptive pill
OH	Orthostatic hypotension
PAF	Paroxysmal atrial fibrillation
PCI	Percutaneous coronary intervention
PCWP	Pulmonary capillary wedge pressure
PDA	Patent ductus arteriosus
PE	Pulmonary embolism
PEEP	Positive end expiratory pressure
PFO	Patent foramen ovale
PICC	Peripherally inserted central catheter
PISA	Proximal isovelocity surface area
PND	Paroxysmal nocturnal dyspnoea
PPM	Permanent pacemaker
RAD	Right axis deviation
RALES	Randomised Aldactone Evaluation Study
RAS	Renal artery stenosis
RBBB	Right bundle branch block
RCA	Right coronary artery
RFA	Radio-frequency ablation
RV	Right ventricle
RWMA	Regional wall motion abnormality
SBE	Subacute bacterial endocarditis
SBP	Systolic blood pressure
SLE	Systemic lupus erythematosus
SOB	Shortness of breath
SpO$_2$	Oxygen saturations
SR	Sinus rhythm
STEMI	ST elevation myocardial infarction
SVC	Superior vena cava
SVT	Supraventricular tachycardia
TFT	Thyroid function test
TIA	Transient ischaemic attack
TIMI	Thrombolysis in myocardial infarction
TOE	Trans-oesophageal echocardiography
TPHT	Treponema pallidum haemagglutination test
TTE	Transthoracic echocardiography
UA	Unstable angina
U&E	Urea and electrolytes

UKPDS	United Kingdom Prospective Diabetes Study
ULSE	Upper left sternal edge
USS	Ultrasound scan
VDRL	Venereal Disease Research Laboratory
VF	Ventricular fibrillation
VQ	Ventilation/perfusion ratio
VSD	Ventricular septal defect
VT	Ventricular tachycardia
WCC	White cell count
WPW	Wolff–Parkinson–White syndrome

Targeted cardiovascular examination

General appearance

The 'end of the bed test' is essential. Does the patient look well or unwell? If they look unwell, it is important to assess them according to the ABC format.

Follow the usual order of inspection, palpation, percussion and finally auscultation, but think logically about underlying diagnoses rather than just going through the routine.

Vital signs

Pulse, blood pressure, temperature and oxygen saturations will often be available before you examine the patient. Observe for signs of haemodynamic compromise. Weight is an important factor for patients with heart failure, and should therefore be measured before breakfast every day to look for a trend.

Peripheral stigmata of cardiovascular disease

Is the patient comfortable? Consider their position. Are they breathless, in pain, coughing or cyanosed? Do they have a normal body habitus?

Hands

- Tar staining indicates that the patient smokes.
- Finger clubbing and central cyanosis are associated with congenital heart disease. Clubbing may also be seen in endocarditis.
- Looks for signs of hyperlipidaemia.

TABLE 1.1 Vital signs and their diagnostic considerations

Bradycardia	< 60 beats/min	MI, conduction disease, drug induced, hypothyroidism, hypothermia
Tachycardia	> 100 beats/min	Sepsis, arrhythmia, heart failure, pulmonary embolus
Hypotension	< 100 mmHg	Low cardiac output heart failure, sepsis, tamponade
Hypertension	> 180 mmHg	Undiagnosed hypertension, coarctation, pain, Conn's syndrome (hyperaldosteronism)
Wide pulse pressure	e.g. 180/80 mmHg	Aortic regurgitation, thyrotoxicosis, atherosclerosis
Narrow pulse pressure	e.g. 110/90 mmHg	Aortic stenosis, congestive heart failure
Low oxygen saturations	< 95%	Lung disease (COPD, interstitial lung disease), heart disease (pulmonary oedema) or both, with VQ mismatch (pulmonary emboli, cardiac shunting)
Fever/pyrexia	> 37.5 °C	Post MI, infective endocarditis

- Signs of infective endocarditis are common if you look carefully. They include:
  — splinter haemorrhages (black streaks under the fingernails)
  — Janeway lesions (painless macular lesions on the palms or soles)
  — Osler's nodes (painful red lesions, usually on the pulps of the fingers and toes).

Face
- Central cyanosis (pulmonary hypertension, intra-cardiac shunt).
- Signs of hyperlipidaemia – xanthelasma are soft yellow plaques around the eyelids, which are associated with lipid disorders.
- Poor dentition predisposes to endocarditis in patients at risk. It is also associated with ischaemic heart disease.

Scars
These often provide a clue to the type of previous surgery.
- Midline sternotomy – any cardiac or thoracic surgery. In the case of CABG, look for where the grafts have come from (saphenous veins, radial arteries).
- Subclavicular – devices (pacemaker, ICD).
- Neck – carotid endarterectomy, although increasingly this is an endovascular procedure (i.e. there is no scar).

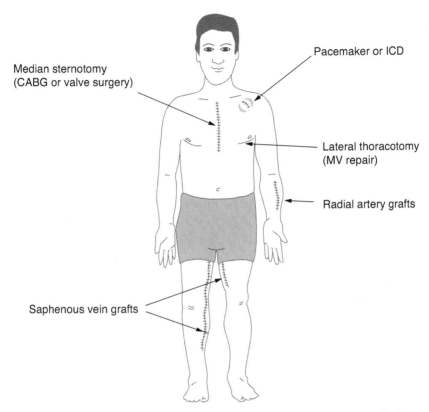

Median sternotomy
(CABG or valve surgery)

Pacemaker or ICD

Lateral thoracotomy
(MV repair)

Radial artery grafts

Saphenous vein grafts

FIGURE 1.1 Schematic diagram of typical surgical scars in the cardiac patient.

Cardiovascular examination

Pulse

Note the rate, rhythm and character. Feel the foot pulses. Are they present and equal? If not, consider peripheral vascular disease, coarctation or aortic dissection.

Blood pressure

Record this from the left and right arm if you suspect dissection or coarctation.

Apex beat

LV enlargement pushes the apex down and out, making it harder to feel. RV enlargement brings the apex closer to the chest wall, creating a 'heaving' character.

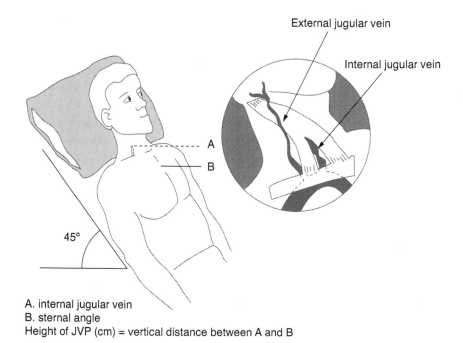

A. internal jugular vein
B. sternal angle
Height of JVP (cm) = vertical distance between A and B

FIGURE 1.2 Assessing the jugular venous pressure.

Jugular venous pressure (JVP)

Look for obvious pulsations at the neck. Distinguish the JVP from the carotid pulse by its double waveform or by obliterating it with gentle compression. Conditions that can be diagnosed from the JVP include the following:

- heart failure
- tricuspid regurgitation (prominent 'v' wave)
- heart block (cannon waves – intermittent large 'a' waves)
- pulmonary hypertension (prominent 'a' wave)
- constrictive pericarditis (paradoxical fall in JVP on inspiration).

Heart sounds and murmurs

Listen for additional heart sounds as well as the loudness of each heart sound. It is important to detect severe valve lesions. In which position is it loudest? Is it systolic or diastolic? This will be covered in more detail later, but typical findings are as follows:

- **Aortic stenosis:** ejection systolic murmur radiating to the carotids. A quiet S2 and narrow pulse pressure indicates severe stenosis.

- **Aortic regurgitation:** early diastolic murmur at the ULSE. If severe, it can be heard at the upper right sternal edge as well.
- **Mitral stenosis:** diastolic murmur at the apex.
- **Mitral regurgitation:** pansystolic murmur audible into the axilla.
- **Tricuspid regurgitation:** pansystolic murmur at the ULSE, raised JVP, and pulsatile liver.

Lungs
Always listen to the lung fields for wheeze and crackles.
- Fine inspiratory and expiratory crackles – typical of pulmonary oedema.
- Fine end-inspiratory crackles – pulmonary fibrosis (check whether the patient is on amiodarone).
- Wheeze – asthma or heart failure.

Ensure that you percuss for pleural effusions, which may occur in the presence of heart failure.

Abdomen
Feel for an enlarged liver in right heart failure or tricuspid regurgitation (when it may be pulsatile). A splenic tip may be palpable in the context of endocarditis. Feel for an abdominal aortic aneurysm.

Peripheral oedema
Check the extent of oedema (e.g. ascertain whether there is sacral or perineal oedema). Consider other causes of lower limb swelling, including lymphatic or venous obstruction, low albumin levels or pelvic obstruction.

Vascular system
Ischaemic heart disease is closely linked to other atherosclerotic diseases, such as peripheral vascular disease, cerebrovascular disease and renovascular disease. Be aware that other systems may be affected when examining and taking a history. For example, if a patient presents with 'new' atrial fibrillation, consider peripheral embolisation, TIA or stroke, and bowel ischaemia.

2

Assessing the patient with chest pain, shortness of breath, syncope and palpitations

Chest pain

It is a medical school cliché that 80% of diagnoses can be made through history taking. But remember that clichés are often true for a reason. History taking is a skill that cannot be fully learned through textbooks, but is refined by many hours of practice with patients. The questions below are intended to serve as a guide and platform for a comprehensive history of chest pain. Particular questions are tailored to help to rule specific diagnoses in or out.

It is important to consider language and cultural differences which may influence the information obtained. Remember that diabetic patients and the elderly may not describe classical symptoms of ischaemia.

History of presenting complaint

- **When did your pain start?**
  Timing is particularly important in the context of STEMI, as it will influence the management and prognosis. This is a medical emergency.
- **Can you describe the pain?**
  Ischaemic pain is classically described as a heavy pain or tightness, like a band around the chest.
- **Where is the pain?**
  Ischaemic pain is classically central or left sided. Other locations (e.g. epigastric or interscapular) are possible. If the pain can be localised with

one finger it is unlikely to be coronary, but remember that ischaemic pain can present in an atypical fashion.

● **Does it radiate anywhere?**
Ischaemic pain classically radiates to the left arm, neck or jaw. Aortic dissection is classically described as a tearing pain between the scapulae, which is maximal at onset. Peptic pain may radiate through to the back.

● **Are there any exacerbating factors?**
Ask about the relationship of the pain to posture, movement and exercise (if possible). Ischaemic pain may be exacerbated by anything that increases myocardial oxygen consumption.

The pain of pulmonary embolism is often made worse by deep inspiration. Pleuritic pain is worsened by anything that causes the pleura to rub against one another. Movement will exacerbate musculoskeletal chest pain.

● **Are there any relieving factors?**
Relieving factors for ischaemia can include nitrates, aspirin, oxygen or opiates. Pericarditic pain is classically relieved by sitting forward.

● **Have you ever had this pain before?**
If the patient has experienced this pain previously, try to gauge whether this is similar or different, and any previous diagnoses that have been made.

● **How severe is the pain?**
Ask the patient to quantify the pain on a scale of 1 to 10, where 10 is 'childbirth' or 'the worst pain you've ever had.'

● **How did it start (suddenly or gradually), and what were you doing at the time of onset?**
Pain related to aortic dissection, MI, embolism or tachyarrhythmia often starts suddenly, whereas that related to unstable angina, pericarditis and pleurisy often starts more gradually.

● **Was the pain at its worst when it first came on?**
Aortic dissection pain is often maximal at onset and may then gradually recede, in contrast to ischaemic pain, which classically increases in a crescendo pattern.

● **Are there any associated symptoms?**
Breathlessness, sweating and nausea are non-specific symptoms but should be documented. Any central or peripheral neurological symptoms may be associated with emboli or dissection.

● **Is the pain constant or intermittent?**
Long-standing, constant pain is less likely to be ischaemic.

● **Would it be painful if I pressed on your chest?**
This is more likely with musculoskeletal chest pain.

Risk factors

It is important to ask about risk factors, but remember that coronary artery disease is possible even in the absence of risk factors.

Direct questions about risk factors for coronary artery disease should ascertain the following:

- advancing age, male gender and ethnicity (high prevalence in South East Asians)
- diabetes – if present, determine whether this is type 1 or 2, its duration, the presence of known micro/macrovascular complications, and the current treatment regimen
- hypertension – if present, ascertain whether it is treated or untreated, the presence of any complications, when the diagnosis was made, and the aetiology if known
- smoking – establish whether this is current or there is a previous history, and determine the pack-year history
- dyslipidaemia – the current lipid profile/cholesterol level must be determined
- family history of premature (age < 45 years) coronary disease – if so, determine in whom, the age at diagnosis, and whether or not they were a smoker
- cocaine use – be tactful when asking about illicit drug use.

If there is a history of known coronary artery disease, it is important to ascertain the following:

- Have they been taking aspirin +/– clopidogrel as prescribed? (risk of stent thrombosis).
- Has the patient had an angiogram or other investigation? If so, where was this performed and what was the result?
- Has the patient had PCI or CABG?
- If there is a history of previous CABG, how many grafts were made and which vessels were grafted? It is useful to get hold of the operation note or previous angiogram reports if you can.

Further questions

You must ask about factors pertaining to procedural risk, so that you are aware of any complications resulting from:

- renal impairment
- peripheral vascular disease (this may influence the site of vascular puncture for the angiogram)
- known aortic disease (including previous surgical intervention or grafting)

- ability to consent
- bleeding risk.

The following are relevant to urgent treatment of STEMI:
- previous haemorrhagic stroke
- embolic stroke in the previous 6 months
- central nervous system trauma or neoplasm
- major trauma, surgery or head injury in the previous 3 weeks
- gastrointestinal bleeding within the last month
- known bleeding disorder
- aortic dissection
- non-compressible puncture (liver biopsy, lumbar puncture)
- transient ischaemic attack within the previous 6 months
- oral anticoagulant therapy
- pregnancy or within 1 week postpartum
- refractory hypertension (systolic blood pressure >180 mmHg, diastolic blood pressure >110 mmHg)
- advanced liver disease
- infective endocarditis
- active peptic ulcer
- refractory resuscitation.

Direct questions should be asked about the following in order to elicit risk factors for other, non-coronary causes of chest pain:
- any regular use of aspirin, NSAIDS or steroids – peptic ulcer disease
- excess alcohol consumption – peptic ulcer disease, pancreatitis
- any recent flights, immobility or cancer – pulmonary embolism
- ask whether the patient has noticed any swelling or pain in their calves – DVT and subsequent embolism
- ask whether the patient is coughing up any sputum – pneumonia with or without complication
- any pain anywhere else.

If the most likely diagnosis is coronary ischaemia, the doctor should ask the following questions related to any contraindications to emergency angioplasty, thrombolysis or other drug treatments:
- Have you ever had a stroke?
- Do you have any bleeding problems, or have you ever been anaemic?
- Do you have a history of renal impairment?

The remainder of the history should be taken in the standard way:

- Do you have any other past medical history?
- Have you ever had an operation?
- Have you had any other hospital appointments, or is your GP treating you for anything?
- Medication – if the patient is describing angina, are they on any treatment and could this be optimised? Is there a reason why they cannot have a beta-blocker (e.g. asthma)?
- Allergies – ask specifically about contrast media, iodine and shellfish allergies if the patient is likely to require coronary angiography (an allergy to shellfish increases the risk of a reaction to iodinated contrast media).
- Family history.
- Social history.
- Systemic enquiry.

Breathlessness

Breathlessness can have a wide variety of causes. The cardiac causes of dyspnoea which must be considered when assessing a patient can be divided into the following groups, although clearly there may be some overlap:

- heart failure due to any cause
- primary heart muscle disorder – hypertrophic, dilated, restrictive and constrictive cardiomyopathy
- valvular causes – any significant valve lesion may cause dyspnoea
- structural heart disease – grown-up congenital heart disease/shunts
- arrhythmias
- pulmonary hypertension (primary or secondary).

The history and examination should be targeted to discern between these possibilities. The following list of screening questions is useful for determining cardiac causes of breathlessness. If a primary respiratory cause is suspected, additional questions should be asked.

History of presenting complaint

- **How long have you been breathless?**
  Acute breathlessness can be associated with myocardial infarction, pulmonary embolism or acute valvular lesion (e.g. mitral chordal rupture). Chronic breathlessness is more likely to be associated with lung disease or heart failure of any cause.

- **Are your symptoms progressive?**
  Chronic heart failure, valvular heart disease and heart muscle disease tend to progress slowly (over many years), whereas acute ischaemia and embolism progress more quickly.
- **Are you more short of breath when lying flat?**
  This suggests left heart failure. Ask the patient about the number of pillows they use when sleeping, and any symptoms of PND.
- **Do you have a cough? If so, is it dry or productive?**
  A dry cough can be associated with heart failure, so remember to ask about ACEi therapy. Productive cough is more common with respiratory disease.
- **Have you ever smoked?**
  Smoking is a risk factor for cardiac ischaemia and respiratory disease.
- **Does your breathlessness come on suddenly?**
- **Have you had any relevant occupational exposure?**
  Examples include industrial toxins that cause cardiomyopathy, or exposure to allergens that cause asthma.
- **Do you have any associated symptoms?**
  Ankle swelling is more common with heart failure. Palpitations are associated with arrhythmia. Chest pain is associated with ischaemia, valvular heart disease and heart muscle disease.

Past medical history/further questions

It is imperative that previous diagnoses of breathlessness (e.g. known valvular heart disease) are recorded, as this may be an acute exacerbation of a chronic condition. If the patient has known heart failure, ask how many hospital admissions they have had previously, and enquire about any weight gain, change in medications, etc. In the context of STEMI/unstable angina causing breathlessness, remember that if a patient cannot lie flat for at least an hour (e.g. with pulmonary oedema), they are unlikely to be able to tolerate an angiogram. This must be treated *before* they reach a catheter lab.

Syncope

Cardiac syncope classically:
- occurs without warning
- may be associated with palpitations
- is associated with a quick recovery following the episode
- is not associated with seizure activity (tongue biting/tonic–clonic fits).

Causes include:
- brady- or tachyarrythmia
- severe valvular heart disease, particularly aortic stenosis
- hypertrophic obstructive cardiomyopathy
- vasovagal response
- carotid sinus syncope
- post-micturition, particularly in male patients.

The history should include the following points:
- any known cardiac disease
- the situation in which the syncope occurred – timing, location, activity at the time, any obvious trigger, and postural changes
- ideally a witness statement should be documented
- single or recurrent episodes
- frequency of symptoms
- associated pre-syncope
- any prodrome, warning symptoms
- how long it took to recover
- associated palpitations (fast/slow, regular/irregular)
- any injuries sustained during syncope – if the patient sustained head or facial injuries, strongly recommend that they are admitted to hospital for investigations
- any suggestion of seizure activity (e.g. tongue biting, urinary incontinence).

Palpitations

History of presenting complaint
- **Was the onset abrupt or gradual?**
  A very abrupt onset is more common with SVT/VT.
- **What was the duration of palpitations?**
  A very short duration (e.g. seconds) is more likely to represent ectopy. Palpitations of very prolonged duration (e.g. several hours to days) are more likely to be atrial fibrillation, and much less likely to be haemodynamically significant. Patients can often be vague, and it is important to be as precise as possible.
- **What was the perceived heart rate at the time?**
  Ask the patient to tap out the rate on the table for you to get an idea of the rate.

- **Were the palpitations regular or irregular?**
  Irregularity is more likely to represent atrial fibrillation.
- **How frequently does the patient have symptoms?**
  This will influence the choice of investigation as outlined above. If a patient only experiences symptoms at night when in bed, this often represents a simple awareness of heartbeat.
- **Are there any associated features?**
  SOB, chest pain, dizziness, nausea and syncope should all be taken seriously and investigated.
- **Is there a history of endocrine disease?**
  Thyroid disease increases the likelihood of arrhythmias.
- **Is there any obvious trigger?**
  For example, exercise, caffeine and alcohol all increase the risk of arrhythmia.
  Caffeine and alcohol intake should be documented. Sudden neck movements or tight collars are associated with carotid sinus hypersensitivity.
- **Is there a history of known cardiac disease?**
- **Is the patient pregnant?**
  Arrhythmia is common in pregnancy.

Investigations

A wide variety of investigations are available for cardiac complaints. It is important to take care when deciding on appropriate investigations to request. Before making such a request, ask yourself what you are trying to find, and what the investigation will add to this. All too commonly a barrage of investigations are requested, many of which are inappropriate.

The table below provides a simple structure for investigations that are likely to yield important information. However, these must not be interpreted rigidly as the rules for investigation of each complaint. For example, a patient may have been admitted with syncope and found to have runs of VT. It may then be appropriate to organise a coronary angiogram to assess the possibility of ischaemia-induced VT. However, you may also wish to perform an echocardiogram looking for specific forms of structural heart disease, which can also result in VT.

Bloods tests can help to exclude biochemical abnormalities, including thyroid dysfunction and electrolyte imbalance, which can predispose to arrhythmia, and anaemia, which may increase the likelihood of syncope. Be selective about the blood investigations that you request, rather than requesting everything in the hope that something will be abnormal.

TABLE 2.1 Relevant investigations

	CHEST PAIN	SHORTNESS OF BREATH	PALPITATIONS	SYNCOPE
ECG	✓	✓	✓	✓
Bloods	Troponin CK-MB	BNP FBC	TFT U&E Magnesium Calcium, phosphate	Troponin CK-MB FBC
Chest X-ray	✓	✓	✗	✗
Echocardiogram	✓	✓	✗	✗
Coronary angiography	✓	✓	✗	✗
Tilt-table testing	✗	✗	✗	✓
Exercise ECG	✓	✗	✓	✓

Cardiac monitors

Although it is often a reflex action to book a 24-hour Holter monitor, it should be remembered that a diagnosis is unlikely to be made if the symptoms are very infrequent. Many cardiologists now consider this to be an unnecessary investigation. Check before booking automatically. Longer periods of Holter monitoring (e.g. 2, 5 and 7 days) are available, or a cardiac memo which the patient activates him- or herself.

Loop recorder (Reveal® device) implantation has proved to be cost-effective in cases with a high index of suspicion of cardiac arrhythmogenic syncope, which are infrequent. These devices are about the size of a memory stick, and are inserted under local anaesthetic in the pre-pectoral region. The patient is then able to trigger the device when they have symptoms, and the recorder can be wirelessly interrogated in hospital. The batteries can last for up to three years.

3

Successful ward rounds in cardiology

Preparation and organisation are the cornerstones to achieving a successful ward round. However, more than this is required in order to provide the best possible care for the patient. Your consultant will be delighted if you are able to competently organise a ward round, but will not be very impressed if you send a patient for a stent without starting aspirin and clopidogrel.

Time management

Time management is an important aspect of any doctor's working life, and a skill that should be learned early on in your career. It encompasses the ability to organise, plan, prioritise and budget time to work effectively and increase productivity. This is especially important in the context of a ward round, as it may have direct ramifications for patient care.

There are several key areas on which you need to focus. It is important to bear these points in mind when doing any ward round, whether it is a consultant or registrar round, or your own ward round.

Up-to-date patient list

It is easy to adopt a lackadaisical approach to producing a patient list, but this will only make your own life more difficult. The following important information should be included on your patient list:
- patient details (name, date of birth and hospital number)
- ward number
- bed number
- admission complaint and past medical history

- current problems and management
- relevant recent blood results, particularly if the patient is anaemic, has renal impairment or is on warfarin
- jobs, including investigations to book, results to chase, etc.

Who to review first

It is tempting to review all of the easy patients first, and leave the more complex ones to concentrate on later. However, you should always see the sickest patients first. This will mean that any potential problems will be recognised earlier in the day, leaving more time in which to contact the relevant people in an attempt to rectify the situation. It is best to categorise patients into one of the three groups listed below, and see them in the following order:

1 sickest patients
2 new patients – as you have never met the patients in this group, you will not know anything about their general condition. They are also likely to require investigative and management plans, which can be complex and time consuming to arrange
3 stable patients – this patient group should be further subdivided as follows:
    - stable but requiring further treatment
    - medically fit for discharge – there is often pressure to see those who can go home early on in the day.

Investigations and procedures

Once the decision has been made to request an investigation or procedure, and depending on what is being requested, it may take some time to organise. Bearing this in mind, the sooner it is requested, the more quickly it is likely to happen. For example, if it is decided at 10 am on a ward round that a patient requires a CT scan, fill in the form at the time and hand it in as soon as possible. If you finish the ward round, go off for lunch and finally hand in the request at 3 pm, it is highly unlikely that the scan will take place that day. At best it will be done the following day. You may find that the scan could have been done on the same day if the request had been handed in earlier. The end result will involve prolonging patient care and lengthening their hospital stay. If more than one junior doctor is present on the round, it may be possible for some urgent jobs to be done by one person while the other continues with the team.

When going to departments to request investigations and procedures, ask yourself whether they are urgent or non-urgent. If they are urgent, always go and discuss them with the relevant person who will actually be performing the investigation or procedure. Not only is this a matter of common courtesy, but also you may be able to negotiate for your investigation or procedure to be performed sooner. Other important factors to bear in mind when making your request include the following:

- Understand what you are requesting.
- Understand what you are trying to prove or disprove. If you are not sure, ask your seniors before making the request. Saying, 'My consultant wanted me to ask for this scan' never goes down particularly well!
- Is what you are requesting appropriate, or even possible? If you are requesting a non-urgent gastroscopy for a patient who has had a troponin-positive cardiac event 3 days previously, your request will be refused. This is because a non-urgent gastroscopy must be performed at least 6 weeks after a troponin-positive cardiac event.
- Has the patient had the appropriate preparation (e.g. nil by mouth or pre-medication)?

Discharge summaries

There is no reason why a discharge summary cannot be started upon admission of the patient. Throughout their admission it can be updated, and this will avoid the last-minute panic of rushing to prepare a poor-quality discharge summary 10 minutes before transport services are due to collect the patient to take them home. Discharge summaries are extremely important as they provide the GP with vital information about the admission, and are a useful source of information when the patient returns to outpatients, or if they end up in Accident and Emergency, where a good background history is extremely valuable.

Working relationships

Medicine is fully established as a multi-disciplinary environment where many different health professionals work together to provide a high quality of care for the patient. In the context of cardiology, the multi-disciplinary team (MDT) is extensive and includes the following:

- doctors (consultant, registrar, junior doctors)
- nursing staff
- specialist nurses (heart failure, chest pain, etc.)
- pharmacists
- cardiac physiologists (echocardiography, exercise tolerance testing)
- radiologists (cardiac CT, cardiac MR, nuclear perfusion scanning)

- physiotherapists
- social workers
- occupational therapists
- bed managers
- secretaries.

It is important to recognise each individual's role and contribution to the team, and the importance that this has for providing high-quality patient care. When you start out as a newly qualified or junior doctor, it is important to recognise that many senior nursing staff have considerable clinical experience. As a result, their knowledge and skills will prove invaluable. Don't turn up on day one and upset or annoy them, as this will only make your own life more difficult.

When you start, you should introduce yourself to the various members of the MDT and make a point of remembering their names. This will make you more approachable, and will also prove beneficial when you are trying to organise investigations or get help. People will be more willing to stay on a few minutes at the end of the day to squeeze your patient on to their list if you are polite and have built up a good rapport with them. A great deal of this may seem obvious, but it is surprising how often it is forgotten or overlooked.

Presenting on ward rounds

Presenting a patient on a ward round involves more than just reading from the notes. More often than not, consultant ward rounds take place on a pre-organised day and at a pre-arranged time, so there should be no excuse for being unprepared.

Preparing for the ward round

You should start to prepare for the ward round about an hour before it begins. This allows plenty of time to get everything ready. A good-quality ward round is one in which you, as the junior, lead your team round the patients, presenting them as you go. We shall break down the process of preparation into categories, each of which is described below.

Patient list

Make sure that you have an up-to-date patient list (as discussed previously), and print off enough copies for everyone who will be on the ward round. Remember to prioritise the order in which the patients are seen!

Bloods folder

- A flow-sheet of blood results from admission is essential. Make sure that this is up to date with the latest results. It is often best to do this before you leave work the previous day, as you must always see blood results on the same day that they are requested. If the results are not going to be back by the time you finish work, hand them over to the on-call doctor to check, together with a plan.
- If a patient is anaemic, look back to see whether this is a new or old finding, and whether it has been appropriately investigated.
- Many patients with cardiovascular disease will also have renovascular disease, so their renal function may be impaired. Ascertain whether this is a new or old finding, and what their baseline level of renal function is like. Renal function can have serious implications for drug dosing, and for investigations and procedures that require the use of contrast media.

Results

Search on the computers and through the old notes for any recent and old investigations and procedures that the patient has had which are relevant to their current admission. Ensure that you read through the results so that you can present them on the ward round. If you don't understand all of the findings, don't be afraid to ask – this shows that you are interested.

Old letters

Old clinic letters provide a vast amount of information about care that the patient has previously received. They can also provide information about other consultants to whom the patient is known, and the management that they are receiving from them. In addition, old letters can be important in the context of further management, investigations and the ceiling of care if appropriate.

New patients

Read through the notes of the new patients to find out the reason for admission, what the management plan is, and what has been done to date. It may also be worth 'eyeballing' the patients from the end of the bed to get a rough idea of their general condition.

Old notes

Old notes provide extremely useful information. However, it can often be difficult to get hold of them. As soon as a patient is admitted, it is worth speaking to the ward clerk to ask them to request the old notes. This will minimise any delays in obtaining them.

Charts

If it is practicable, before the ward round is due to start, go round all of your patients and open the observation charts and drug charts at the end of the bed so that they are ready for the consultant to review. If you are running about trying to track down where the charts have gone, not only does this waste time but also it looks unprofessional.

Preparing patients for permanent pacemakers and percutaneous coronary intervention

It is not uncommon for patients to be sent for procedures having had inadequate preparation. This may result in the cancellation of the proposed procedure, and a delay in patient care. Most hospitals will have a protocol available from the department or on the intranet. It is worth looking at this to ensure that you have fully complied with it. Some protocols will mention a 'signed consent form.' However, unless you can actually perform the procedure yourself, do not fill this in. You should not consent patients for a procedure that you are unable to perform, as you are unlikely to fully understand or be able to convey to the patient the risks involved.

Ensure that the patient is aware of the proposed procedure, and that before they arrive in the department they understand the procedure and agree to it being done. The written consent form can be dealt with by the health professional who will be performing the procedure.

Permanent pacemakers (PPM)

- Routine investigations prior to PPM insertion (these investigations should also be repeated after the procedure):
  - bloods – FBC, U&E, clotting screen, group and save
  - MRSA screen
  - chest X-ray
  - 12-lead ECG.
- If the patient is on warfarin, this should usually be discontinued for 4 days prior to the insertion of the PPM, unless otherwise stated by a cardiology consultant.
- It is debatable whether patients can remain on aspirin, but clopidogrel should usually be discontinued. You should check with the physician or department that will be inserting the PPM whether they would like the

aspirin or clopidogrel to be stopped. Remember that clopidogrel needs to be discontinued for at least 1 week to ensure that its effects have worn off.

- Ensure that your patient has peripheral venous access before they are sent to have their pacemaker inserted. This provides a route for administering sedation, a safety net in the event of any complications, and may be used to administer contrast to determine venous anatomy. For the last reason it should therefore be placed on the patient's left side, assuming that a left-sided implant is planned.

- Antibiotic prophylaxis – consult with your local hospital guidelines, as these may vary. Commonly the antibiotic of choice is gentamicin 80 mg IV plus co-amoxiclav 1.2 g IV at induction. In penicillin-allergic patients clarithromycin may be used as an alternative to co-amoxiclav and vancomycin, if the patient is at risk of MRSA. If in doubt check with the microbiologist.

- Post-procedure:
  - Check the wound for local swelling, bleeding and haematoma formation. Do not remove any dressings, but merely add to them if necessary. This will reduce the risk of infection.
  - Auscultate and percuss the chest to rule out a clinically significant pneumothorax if the patient has suggestive symptoms.
  - Listen to the heart sounds and inspect the JVP to rule out pericardial effusion/tamponade if indicated.
  - ECG – remember that, depending on the indication, this may not necessarily show pacing spikes.
  - Chest X-ray – PA and lateral views will help to assess lead position and rule out a subclinical pneumothorax.
  - Pacing check – this will usually be performed on the day of the procedure, or on the following day if the implantation was late in the day. It will be repeated 6 weeks later, and is often organised by the pacing department.

Percutaneous coronary intervention (PCI)

- Routine investigations prior to PCI (with the exception of group and save, these investigations should also be repeated after the procedure):
  - bloods – FBC, U&E (important in the context of contrast nephropathy), clotting screen, group and save, troponin in the case of acute MI or unstable angina
  - chest X-ray
  - 12-lead ECG.

- Check with the patient whether they have any known allergies to contrast media or dyes, latex, iodine or shellfish, and that they are not at risk of contrast nephropathy. If they are, they may need hydrocortisone and chlorpheniramine IV before the procedure.
- Loading doses of drugs pre-procedure:
  — Aspirin 300 mg.
  — Clopidogrel – patients who are already taking clopidogrel 75 mg per day do not need loading unless the consultant indicates otherwise. Patients not previously on clopidogrel should have 300 mg clopidogrel the day before or 600 mg on the day of the procedure. Loading doses should be checked with the operating consultant.
  — Glycoprotein IIb/IIIa drugs may be indicated in the context of acute myocardial infarction (*see* Chapter 4).
  — If the patient has been receiving LMWH for NSTEMI or unstable angina, the morning dose is usually omitted (and IV heparin can be given in the cath lab). This prevents unnecessary bleeding complications when obtaining arterial access.
- If the patient is on warfarin already, discuss this with your seniors. There are important implications with regard to haemorrhage risk, especially in the context of loading the patient on aspirin and clopidogrel.
- Metformin:
  — Metformin should be stopped 3 days prior to coronary angiography (X-ray contrast can impair metformin excretion and lead to development of a lactic acidosis).
  — Renal function must be checked 48 hours post-procedure. If the creatinine level is still at the baseline value, metformin can safely be restarted. If the creatinine level is raised from the baseline value, renal function must be monitored before restarting the metformin. Monitor the blood sugar levels and be prepared to start a sliding scale in some cases.
- Post-procedure:
  — If the patient has stents inserted, or has suffered an MI, they must remain on clopidogrel for 1 year, and on aspirin for life.
  — Check the puncture site (radial or femoral) for bleeding, bruising, haematoma and pseudoaneurysm formation.
  — Palpate the distal pulses and ensure that the limb is neurovascularly intact.
  — Examine the respiratory and cardiovascular systems to rule out pneumothorax and pericardial effusion/tamponade.

— Perform an ECG (and compare with that pre-procedure).
— Repeat bloods (FBC, U&E and troponin) the following day in high-risk patients and those at risk of contrast nephropathy. However, maximal renal insult will occur approximately 5 days post-contrast, so if this is anticipated, steps should be taken to check U&E on day 5, and the results should be communicated to the team.

Work-up for heart valve replacement

Although there have been great advances in cardiac surgery over the years, it is not without complications. Of these, perhaps one of the most feared is an infected prosthetic valve. Therefore these patients require a meticulous work-up prior to valve replacement.

A variety of different replacement valve options exist. Although the choice of valve will be decided by the consultant surgeon, it is advisable to have an understanding of the main types of valve (*see* Figure 3.1):

- Starr–Edwards valve – caged-ball valve (old, and rarely used now except in cases of redo valve surgery)
- St Jude valve – bileaflet valve
- Bjork–Shiley and Medtronic Hall – tilting-disc valves
- xenograft tissue valve – these patients will not require lifelong anticoagulation treatment
- transcatheter aortic valve implantation (TAVI) – this is a relatively new method of 'percutaneous' valve implantation, and it is only performed at specialist centres.

A number of investigations must be undertaken prior to surgery. These are summarised below.

Bloods
- FBC:
  — anaemia
  — infection.
- U&E:
  — renal impairment.
- LFT:
  — mildly deranged LFT may be seen in right heart failure as a result of hepatic congestion.
- Clotting.
- Group and save.
- Blood cultures.

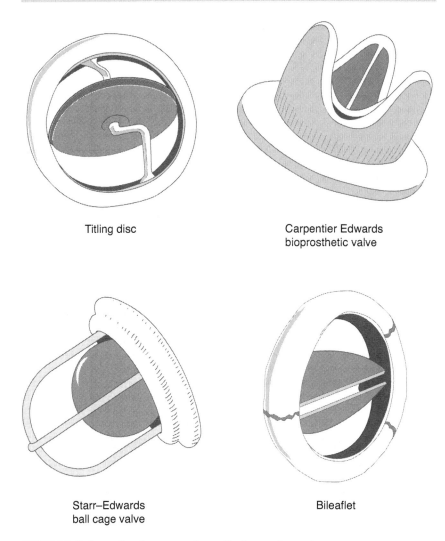

Titling disc

Carpentier Edwards
bioprosthetic valve

Starr–Edwards
ball cage valve

Bileaflet

FIGURE 3.1 Schematic diagrams of prosthetic cardiac valves.

Chest X-ray
- Infection.
- May show signs of heart failure.

Echocardiogram
- Must have a recent echocardiogram, ideally within the last 3 months.

Coronary angiography

- This should be performed in all patients at risk of coronary disease. If there is significant coronary artery disease, this may be 'by-passed' at the same time as valve surgery.

Electrocardiogram

It is especially important to look for evidence of hypertrophic changes and strain patterns. Mitral valve disease frequently results in atrial fibrillation.

Dental review

- Minimise the risk of potential sites for infection of the prosthetic valve.
- Dental extractions may be necessary before cardiac surgery.

Pulmonary function testing

- This is necessary for any major operation, and will form part of the anaesthetic risk assessment.

Work-up for coronary artery by-pass grafting (CABG)

These patients require a very similar work-up, with the exception of the dental review.

Bloods

- FBC:
    - anaemia is an important cause of chest pain and shortness of breath, and must be fully investigated before CABG
    - ensure that the patient does not have a raised WCC indicating an infection prior to surgery.
- U&E:
    - patients with cardiovascular disease will frequently also have renovascular disease, so may commonly have renal impairment.
- Clotting screen.
- Group and save.

Chest X-ray

- Infection.
- May show signs of heart failure.

Echocardiogram

- Assessment of left ventricular ejection fraction.

- Identification of regional wall motion abnormalities. These may be the result of infarcted myocardium. If this is the case, it is important to ensure that this myocardium is viable. This can be done by myocardial perfusion scanning. If the myocardium is not viable, there is little point in proceeding with revascularisation.

Coronary angiography
- Assessment of left ventricular function, although this information should predominantly come from an echocardiogram.
- Angiography will highlight any stenotic lesions within the coronary artery vasculature. This will indicate which areas need to be by-passed in order to achieve revascularisation.

ECG
- There may be ischaemia. The pattern of the ischaemia will help to identify which vessels are responsible.

Pulmonary function testing
- This is necessary for any major operation, and will form part of the anaesthetic risk assessment.

Myocardial perfusion scan (nuclear, MRI or stress echo)
- Assessment of myocardial viability is extremely important prior to revascularisation. If the myocardium is not viable, revascularisation will be of no benefit.

Carotid artery Doppler scan
- In some instances patients may require surgery for carotid artery disease as well as CABG surgery.

Talking to families and patients
This aspect of medicine is often completely overlooked, but is arguably one of the most important areas. Many of us are extremely busy, but this should not prevent us from setting aside time to explain what is happening to both the patient and their family.

Before you discuss any information with a patient you must ascertain what, if anything, they want to know. On occasion you will meet patients who do not wish to know about any aspect of their illness. In all cases you must always gain the patient's consent to any discussion with their family.

Daily updates

A brief update on a daily basis during the ward round is a good way to explain the current plan for the patient, and also to gauge how the patient feels about this. Updating and explaining the results of any investigations and discussing the plan for any further investigations will go a long way towards alleviating the anxiety of both the patient and their family.

After your daily update, ask the patient and their family if they have any questions. This will ensure that everything has been covered. These brief updates are extremely reassuring for patients, and will also help to prevent lengthy discussions with dissatisfied relatives.

Formal discussions

On occasion it is not appropriate to give the patient or their family a brief update on the ward. The classic example is, of course, breaking bad news. In this instance it is important to set time aside. A specific time should be arranged that is convenient for both parties. It is essential that you find a more private area than the open ward. Switch off your bleep and phone, or hand them to a colleague. Take time to discuss any information, and invite questions. After any discussion, it may be appropriate to ask the patient and their family if they would like to remain in the room for a short time after you have left.

Documentation

This is usually very poorly done in practice. Documentation of any discussions will be very useful for ensuring that on-call teams are aware of the current situation and what the patient knows. It can also be extremely important in retrospective medico-legal cases.

Daily updates should be included in the ward-round notes, and need only be brief. Any formal discussions should be clearly documented with the following information:

- date and time of discussion
- the names of all individuals present at the discussion. Document the names of family members, e.g. Jane Smith, rather than just 'sister'. The patient may have four sisters, one of whom is estranged!
- the information given and general level of explanation
- any questions or concerns raised by the patient or their family.

4

Safe prescribing in cardiology

The area of safe prescribing and drug errors is one of particular interest and rapidly growing importance. Many of the drugs used in cardiology have interactions with each other, and there are specific contraindications in certain patient groups. However, these drugs can potentially be of great benefit, although at the cost of being extremely dangerous if they are incorrectly prescribed. We shall not discuss the pharmacology of these drugs, but will focus on the various aspects of safe prescribing and their major implications. In the event of any drug queries, the *British National Formulary* should always be consulted, and this list should not act as a substitute for that resource.

Angiotensin-converting-enzyme inhibitors (ACEi)

Indications
- Blood pressure control (first-line management in patients under 55 years old, but usually not in black patients).
- Prophylaxis for cardiovascular events – within the first 24 hours after myocardial infarction.
- Heart failure.
- All diabetic patients with microalbuminuria.

Contraindications
- Renal failure – check renal function before initiation of the drug, and monitor the patient's response.
- Hypotensive patients (unless there is heart failure and the patient is asymptomatic).
- Known renal artery stenosis – caution is needed, as patients with cardiovascular disease are more likely to have renovascular disease.

Often a test dose consisting of a low-dose ACE inhibitor (e.g. captopril) can be used if you are concerned.
- Pregnancy.

Important notes
- Concomitant use with NSAIDs increases the risk of renal damage.
- Concomitant use with diuretics, especially potassium-sparing drugs, increases the risk of hyperkalaemia.

Adverse effects
- First-dose hypotension.
- Cough, due to breakdown of bradykinin. If this occurs, an angiotensin-2-receptor blocker (A2RB) may be more suitable.
- Renal failure.
- Hyperkalaemia.

Aldosterone antagonists (spironolactone and eplerenone)

Indications
- Left ventricular dysfunction (LVEF ≤ 40%) post myocardial infarction.
- NYHA Class III and IV, although there is increasing evidence that these drugs are useful in all classes of heart failure.

Contraindications
- Hyperkalaemia (> 5.5 mmol/l).
- Renal impairment with creatinine clearance ≤ 30 ml/min.

Adverse effects
- Gynaecomastia (associated with spironolactone).
- Hyperkalaemia.
- Diarrhoea and nausea.
- Hypotension and dizziness.

Amiloride

Indications
- Oedema.
- Potassium conservation (amiloride is a weak diuretic when used alone, and is therefore often combined with a loop or thiazide diuretic).
- Congestive cardiac failure.

Contraindications
- Hyperkalaemia.
- Anuria.

Important notes
- Monitor electrolytes closely when initiating patients on amiloride. This is especially important if the patient is also on an ACEi or A2RB, due to the risk of severe hyperkalaemia.

Adverse effects
- Hyperkalaemia.
- Postural hypotension.
- Gastrointestinal disturbance.

Amiodarone

Indications
- Both supraventricular and ventricular arrhythmias.

Contraindications
- Previous intolerance.
- Pregnancy and breastfeeding.
- Sinus node bradycardia, atrioventricular block, second- and third-degree heart block in individuals without pacemakers.

Important notes
- Amiodarone inhibits the cytochrome P450 enzyme group, and therefore reduces clearance of many other drugs (e.g. digoxin, simvastatin, warfarin). Consider dose reduction when initiating amiodarone.

Adverse effects
- Hyper- and hypothyroidism (hypothyroidism is more common than hyperthyroidism).
- Pulmonary fibrosis.
- Corneal microdeposits.
- Deranged liver function due to drug-induced hepatitis.
- Slate-grey skin discoloration and photosensitivity.
- Dysrhythmias can occur with any anti-arrhythmic drug.

Aspirin

Indications
- Primary and secondary prevention of cardiovascular events.
- Atrial fibrillation.
- Myocarditis (often used in high doses).
- Post-coronary stent or by-pass grafting.

Contraindications
- Allergy or intolerance to aspirin or NSAIDs.
- Current peptic ulcer disease.
- Previous gastrointestinal haemorrhage (discuss with senior colleagues the balance of risks and potential benefits of the drug).

Important notes
- Consider the use of either enteric-coated aspirin or proton pump inhibitors/ H_2-receptor antagonists for gastroprotection.

Adverse effects
- Gastrointestinal erosion and ulcers resulting in gastrointestinal bleeding are relatively common.
- Bleeding.
- Bruising.

Beta-blockers

Indications
- Angina.
- Myocardial infarction.
- Arrhythmias – first-line treatment for atrial fibrillation.
- Heart failure – some beta-blockers reduce mortality in any grade of stable heart failure. There is no clear guidance about what to do in acute heart failure.
- Hypertension – although beta-blockers reduce blood pressure, they have only a limited effect on the reduction of stroke, myocardial infarction and cardiovascular mortality as compared with ACEi, calcium-channel blockers and diuretics.

Contraindications
- Second- or third-degree heart block.

- Worsening or unstable heart failure, or patients with overt heart failure – cardiac output will be reduced.
- Asthma.

Important notes
- Concomitant use with rate-limiting calcium-channel blockers (e.g. verapamil, diltiazem) can result in profound bradycardia and the precipitation of heart failure.

Adverse effects
- Cold peripheries.
- Nightmares and sleep disturbance.
- Erectile dysfunction.
- Bradycardia.
- Depression.

Clopidogrel

Indications
- Secondary prevention after myocardial ischaemia.
- Antiplatelet agent post PCI with stent insertion.

Contraindications
- Active bleeding.

Important notes
- A loading dose of 300 mg should be administered to patients undergoing PCI unless they are already established on treatment. Some centres use a loading dose of 600 mg. However, this is unlicensed.

Adverse effects
- Bleeding.
- Gastrointestinal side-effects (e.g. dyspepsia, abdominal pain, diarrhoea).

Digoxin

Indications
- Supraventricular arrhythmias, particularly AF. Digoxin can be useful in patients with heart failure and AF, or as an adjunct if beta-blockers

or calcium-blockers fail to provide adequate rate control. Digoxin is not so useful for rate control during exercise. Remember to prescribe a loading dose.

- Heart failure – this is an 'add-on' therapy for patients with NYHA Class IV heart failure. It offers symptomatic relief, and one study has shown a decline in hospital admissions, but there is no mortality benefit.

Contraindications
- Second- or third-degree heart block.
- Renal failure – this can quickly lead to digoxin toxicity, so adjust the dose!
- Supraventricular arrhythmias associated with an accessory pathway (e.g. Wolff–Parkinson–White syndrome).

Important notes
- There is an increased incidence of toxicity in patients with hypokalaemia, hypomagnesaemia and hypercalcaemia. If toxicity is suspected, send a blood sample for a digoxin level.

Adverse effects
- Nausea, vomiting, diarrhoea and dizziness are perhaps the most common adverse effects.
- Conduction disturbances.

Enoxaparin
Indications
- DVT prophylaxis in patients at risk during hospital admissions. Dose at 40 mg once daily unless there is renal impairment.
- Post acute NSTEMI/STEMI at 1 mg/kg twice a day.

Contraindications
- Active bleeding, recent cerebral haemorrhage or bleeding diathesis.
- Thrombocytopenia (including previous heparin-induced thrombocytopenia).

Important notes
- Renal impairment – reduce the dose by half in patients with a creatinine clearance of < 30 ml/min.
- Enoxaparin can be used in pregnancy.

Adverse effects
- Haemorrhage.
- Skin necrosis.
- Heparin-induced thrombocytopenia. Suspect this if there is more than a 50% reduction in platelet count, often occurring 5 to 10 days after initiation of heparin in patients with thrombosis, skin necrosis or microemboli.

Flecainide

Indications
- Supraventricular tachycardias (AVNRT and WPW).
- Chemical cardioversion of atrial fibrillation.

Contraindications
- Flecainide should not be used in patients with an abnormal LV, as it may precipitate ventricular arrhythmia.
- Heart failure.
- History of myocardial infarction.
- Sinus node dysfunction, second-degree heart block or greater.

Important notes
- Flecainide should only be administered by people with experience of its use, and should be discussed with a cardiologist.
- Class Ic anti-arrhythmic drug (Vaughan Williams classification of anti-arrhythmic drugs).

Adverse effects
- Arrhythmia, especially in patients with hypokalaemia.
- Fatigue.
- Oedema.

Glycoprotein 2b/3a inhibitors (eptifibatide, tirofiban and abciximab)

Indications
- Prevention of early myocardial infarction in patients with angina or NSTEMI *and* with chest pain within the last 12–24 hours (depending on which drug is used).

Contraindications

- Stroke within the previous 30 days, or any history of haemorrhagic stroke.
- Intracranial pathology (aneurysm, neoplasm or arteriovenous malformation).
- Severe hypertension.
- Haemorrhagic diathesis, increased prothrombin time/INR or thrombocytopenia.
- Extreme caution should be exercised in the following patient groups:
  — prolonged CPR, major surgery or severe trauma within the previous 3 months
  — aortic dissection or puncture of a non-compressible vessel within the previous 24 hours
  — organ biopsy within the previous 2 weeks.

Important notes

- Monitor platelet count, haemoglobin and haematocrit before treatment, 2–6 hours after initiation of treatment, and then at least once daily.

Adverse effects

- Bleeding manifestations – in the case of severe haemorrhage that is uncontrolled by pressure, discontinue treatment immediately.
- Reversible thrombocytopenia.

Ivabradine

Indications

- Add-on therapy for patients with angina where HR is > 60 bpm. Often used in patients who cannot tolerate beta-blockers.

Contraindications

- Severe bradycardia (should not be initiated if heart rate is less than 60 beats per minute).
- Patients not in sinus rhythm.
- Cardiogenic shock.
- Sick sinus syndrome, second-degree heart block or greater, patients with pacemakers.

Important notes

- Ivabradine lowers the heart rate by acting as an I_f-receptor blocker in the sinus node. Therefore the patient must be in sinus rhythm for it to be effective.

Adverse effects
- Bradycardia.
- First-degree heart block.
- Headaches and dizziness.

Loop diuretics (furosemide, bumetanide)

Indications
- Acute or chronic heart failure.
- Can be added to antihypertensive treatments to achieve tighter blood pressure control in cases of resistant hypertension.

Contraindications
- Severe hypokalaemia and hyponatraemia.
- Anuria.

Important notes
- Patients on IV infusions of loop diuretics should have their renal function monitored daily.
- Replace electrolytes as required.
- Furosemide causes hypokalaemia in some patients. Think about the pharmacology rather than just replacing the potassium continuously if the patient is likely to remain on furosemide in the long term. The addition of amiloride or spironolactone (a potassium-sparing diuretic) will help to retain potassium, with the benefit of additional diuresis. Co-amilofruse is a combination drug that contains both furosemide and amiloride.

Adverse effects
- Hypotension and postural hypotension.
- Renal dysfunction and nephrotoxicity.
- Hypokalaemia, hyponatraemia, hypocalcaemia and hypomagnesaemia.

Nicorandil

Indications
- Prophylaxis and treatment of angina.

Contraindications
- LVF with a low filling pressure.
- Hypotension.
- Cardiogenic shock.

Important notes
- Nicorandil acts as a potassium-channel activator and results in arteriovenous dilatation.

Adverse effects
- Headache – this is common on initiation of treatment and may be transient. Warn the patient in advance, in order to aid compliance in the long term.
- Facial flushing due to vasodilatory properties.
- Rarely, oral ulceration has been reported.

Nitrates (isosorbide mononitrate, isosorbide dinitrate, glyceryl trinitrate)

Indications
- Prophylaxis and treatment of angina.
- Acute and congestive cardiac failure (glyceryl trinitrate).

Contraindications
- Hypotension.
- Aortic stenosis.
- Hypertrophic cardiomyopathy.
- Mitral stenosis.

Important notes
- Tolerance may develop unless a nitrate-free period of duration 4–8 hours is maintained.

Adverse effects
- Headache.
- Hypotension and postural hypotension.
- Tachycardia (as well as paradoxical bradycardia).
- Dizziness.

Statins

Indications
- Primary and secondary prevention of cardiovascular disease.
- Hypercholesterolaemia and dyslipidaemia.

Contraindications
- Use with caution in patients with a history of liver disease or high alcohol intake.
- Extreme caution is needed in patients with a history of myositis and rhabdomyolysis.

Important notes
- Monitor liver function before initiating treatment, and also at 3 months and 12 months after initiating treatment.
- Some statins (e.g. atorvastatin) have beneficial effects on triglycerides that other statins do not have. Consult local guidelines and the *British National Formulary* for further information.

Adverse effects
- Myositis, and in severe cases it can lead on to rhabdomyolysis.
- Drug-induced hepatitis.
- Malaise.

Thiazide diuretics (bendroflumethiazide and indapamide)

Indications
- Hypertension.
- Oedema.

Contraindications
- Refractory hypokalaemia, hyponatraemia and hypercalcaemia.
- Symptomatic hyperuricaemia.

Important notes
- Bendroflumethiazide at doses above 2.5 mg has no additional benefit in terms of reducing blood pressure. Increased doses result in more marked changes in potassium, sodium, calcium and uric acid levels, and should therefore be avoided.

Adverse effects
- Hypotension and postural hypotension.
- Electrolyte disturbances – hypokalaemia, hyponatraemia and hypercalcaemia.
- Precipitation of acute gout.

Thrombolytic agents

Indications
- STEMI – patients must have chest pain *plus* ST elevation of ≥ 1 mm in two or more limb leads, or ST elevation of ≥ 2 mm in two or more contiguous chest leads, or new LBBB.
- Onset of pain less than 12 hours previously. May be useful for onset of pain up to 24 hours previously.

Contraindications
- Absolute contraindications – active bleeding, malignancy, aortic dissection, abdominal aortic aneurysm, cerebral haemorrhage (at any time), ischaemic stroke (in the past 6 months), known cerebral aneurysm or arterio-venous malformation (AVM).
- Relative contraindications – severe uncontrolled hypertension (blood pressure $\geq 180/110$ mmHg), current use of anticoagulants, bleeding diathesis, trauma in the past 2–4 weeks, pregnancy, active peptic ulcer disease.

Important notes
- Streptokinase must not be given more than once in any patient's lifetime, due to the formation of antibodies. It will be ineffective and may cause an allergic reaction.
- Primary PCI is superior to thrombolysis and remains the treatment of choice.

Adverse effects
- Severe uncontrolled haemorrhage at any site. Intracerebral haemorrhage is a particularly unfortunate complication.
- Anaphylactic reaction to thrombolytic therapy.

Warfarin

Indications
- Prophylaxis of prosthetic heart valve thrombosis.
- Prophylaxis of embolism in rheumatic heart disease.
- Prophylaxis of venous and arterial thrombosis and embolism.
- Prophylaxis of embolism in atrial fibrillation.
- Treatment of thromboembolic disease.

Contraindications
- Active bleeding.
- Peptic ulcer disease.
- Severe hypertension.
- Anaemia that has not been fully investigated.
- A patient who has suffered recurrent falls or is at significant risk of falls.

Important notes
- Prior to initiation of treatment with warfarin the patient must be counselled.
- The patient must be given a card to carry which states that they are on warfarin, with the indication and duration of treatment and target INR (usually 2–3 except for metal heart valves where it is 3–4).

Adverse effects
- Haemorrhage.
- Rash.
- Skin necrosis.

5

Introduction to specialist investigations

Electrocardiogram

A detailed consideration of specialist investigations is beyond the scope of this book. However, there are some vitally important points that need to be covered. All patients who are admitted to hospital should have a baseline ECG recording, irrespective of their complaint on admission. It is a cheap, simple and non-invasive investigation that can provide a great deal of information.

Recording a brief description of the ECG in a discharge summary can prove particularly useful at a later date, especially in the modern era of electronic discharge summaries. If a patient is readmitted in the future, knowledge of a previous baseline ECG may be potentially life-saving, particularly in the context of a patient presenting acutely with chest pain and an abnormal ECG.

Important measurements

There are certain measurements on an ECG with which you should be familiar. You should be comfortable with the interconversion of these measurements in 'seconds', and 'number of small squares', which is summarised overleaf:

1 small square (i.e. 1 mm) = 0.04 seconds

5 small squares (i.e. 5 mm) = 0.2 seconds.

TABLE 5.1 Normal values

	SECONDS	NUMBER OF SMALL SQUARES
PR interval	0.12–0.20	3–5
QRS duration	0.04–0.12	1–3
QT interval	Male: 0.39 Female: 0.41	Male: 9.75 Female: 10.25

With regard to the QT interval, it is best to work on the average of 0.40 seconds (10 small squares). The QT interval will vary depending on the heart rate, and will increase with bradycardia and decrease with tachycardia. This can be calculated using Bazett's formula to give the *corrected QT interval (QTc)*:

$$QTc = \frac{QT}{\sqrt{RR\ interval}}$$

Voltage criteria for left ventricular hypertrophy

When looking at an ECG, it is possible to 'diagnose' LVH. It is often not a definitive diagnostic investigation, but can alert a clinician to the possibility. The only definitive method of assessing LVH is by imaging. False-positive and false-negative results occur when calculating voltage criteria for LVH in the following situations:

- false-positive results – young slim patients will often have large complexes but no LVH
- false-negative results – obese patients may have a 'normal'-looking ECG, or an ECG with small complexes as a result of increased transthoracic impedance, but actually have LVH.

Several different voltage criteria methods exist, one of the most popular and easiest to apply in clinical practice being the Sokolow–Lyon criteria:

- S in V_1 + R in V_5 or V_6 (whichever is larger) ≥ 35 mm
- R in aVL ≥ 11 mm.

If voltage criteria for LVH are present on the ECG, look for any 'strain' pattern. Strain in the context of LVH indicates that there is insufficient myocardial perfusion. This is a direct result of an increased myocardial bulk, with an unchanged or decreased blood supply from the coronary arteries. On an ECG this is represented by ST depression and T-wave inversion in V4–V6, together with voltage criteria for LVH.

ECG vascular territories

The ECG can provide information about the site of an area of infarct or ischaemia. This can be especially important in the context of the acute management, and also has a bearing on the prognosis. There is some variation in the coronary artery anatomy. However, the following should provide a basic guide to the vascular territory.

Anterior or anteroseptal infarction/ischaemia
- ECG territory – V1–V4.
- Vascular territory – almost always left anterior descending artery.
- Anterior MIs have a worse prognosis than other territories, and frequently result in left ventricular impairment. This group benefits from immediate reperfusion and early pharmacological treatment.

Inferior infarction/ischaemia
- ECG territory – II, III and aVF.
- Vascular territory – usually caused by a lesion of the right coronary artery. However, less commonly it can be caused by a lesion of the circumflex artery.

Lateral infarction/ischaemia
- ECG territory – V5–V6 and/or I and aVL.
- Vascular territory – often caused by a lesion of the circumflex artery, or the diagonal branch of the left anterior descending artery.

Posterior infarction
- ECG territory – ST segment depression in V1–V3 with dominant R-waves, so-called reciprocal changes in the anterior chest leads.
- Vascular territory – most commonly due to right coronary artery lesions, but may be caused by a lesion of the circumflex artery in circumflex dominant patients.

Posterior and right-sided electrocardiogram

In the case of a suspected posterior myocardial infarction, a posterior ECG should be performed. Leads labelled V7–V10 are placed on the chest wall as follows:
- V7 – posterior axillary line
- V8 – halfway between V7 and V9
- V9 – to the left of the spine
- V10 – to the right of the spine.

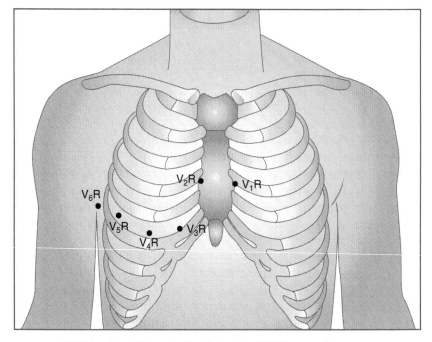

FIGURE 5.1 ECG lead positions for the right-sided ECG recording.

In as many as one-third of patients with a posterior or inferior STEMI, right ventricular infarction may be present. If this is extensive, it may be observed on a 12-lead ECG where ST elevation in V1 is accompanied by inferior or posterior STEMI. A right-sided ECG can be of benefit, and is performed by placing the chest leads in a mirror image layout to those of a normal ECG.

Exercise tolerance testing

Exercise tolerance testing (ETT) is one of several types of cardiac stress test. It is an extremely useful investigation, and moreover it is non-invasive. Despite this, it is only of value in symptomatic patients. Exercise testing in asymptomatic patients has been found to be largely inaccurate, giving high false-positive rates. There tends to be a higher incidence of false-positive results in female patients compared with males.

Within the symptomatic patient group, a positive test result can confirm a clinical diagnosis. However, a negative test result may in fact be a false-negative, and furthermore has a low correlation with the absence of coronary artery disease. As a result, ETT has major limitations with regard to the diagnosis of diseased versus normal coronary arteries.

There are two main types of treadmill ETT that you should be aware of:
1 Bruce protocol
2 modified Bruce protocol.

The Bruce protocol consists of a standardised seven-stage protocol for cardiac stress testing. Each stage is 3 minutes long, and there is a progressively increasing level of difficulty. The modified Bruce protocol is less demanding and more suitable for the elderly or those with limited mobility. This modified protocol can also be useful for risk-stratifying patients with known ischaemic heart disease who present with troponin and ECG-negative chest pain. A negative test aids the planning of discharge.

Considerations when sending a patient for ETT

Many inappropriate requests for ETT are made, some with little consideration of what is involved in the investigation.

- Exercise tolerance – ensure that the patient is able to walk unaided for a reasonable distance or length of time. There is little point in sending an 85-year-old man who mobilises for 100 yards with a walking frame and is limited by his breathing due to COPD.
- Medications – do you want the investigation to be performed with the patient on or off rate-limiting medications such as beta-blockers and calcium-channel blockers?
- Previous ETT – if your patient has had previous ETT, when was their last test, what were the results and do you need to repeat it again? It may be that other investigations are more appropriate.
- Consider whether the Bruce or modified Bruce test is more appropriate.

Indications for ETT

- Diagnosis of coronary artery disease – as discussed previously, the main benefit is found in symptomatic 'high-risk' patients with a high pre-test likelihood of disease.
- Evaluation:
  — assessment of cardiac function and quantification of exercise capacity
  — serial testing to evaluate the effect of medical or surgical intervention.
- Prognosis following myocardial infarction.

- Detection of exercise-induced arrhythmias and arrhythmia syndromes (e.g. long QT syndrome).

Contraindications to ETT

Patients with heart failure need to be carefully considered, as their mobility may be limited by breathing rather than by chest pain. Other forms of cardiac stress test may be more suitable for these types of patients.

The following are contraindications to ETT:

- acute myocardial infarction
- severe aortic stenosis
- acute myocarditis or pericarditis
- acute aortic dissection
- severe left main stem stenosis
- complete heart block
- uncontrolled hypertension.

Normal response to ETT

- Increased ventricular rate – age-adjusted target heart rates can be roughly calculated using the formulae *220 minus age in years* for men, and *210 minus age in years* for women.
- The PR interval shortens.
- The QT interval shortens.
- The R-wave amplitude decreases.
- The ST segment is sharply up-sloping.
- Blood pressure rises.

What constitutes a positive ETT result?

Interpretation of an exercise test can be difficult, and unless you are familiar with this type of investigation you must consult a specialist (i.e. cardiology registrar or consultant).

Chest pain

Chest pain with ST depression strongly suggests a positive ETT. However, chest pain without ECG changes should not be disregarded.

ST depression

- ST depression of ≥ 1 mm is deemed to be significant. Some centres will prefer to use 1.5 or 2.0 mm as a minimum. With these higher values the predictive accuracy increases, although at the expense of sensitivity.
- The measurement of ST depression should be taken 80 ms after the J point.

ST elevation

This may occur in leads that had Q-waves at rest, and it has the same significance as ST depression.

Systolic blood pressure

Failure to mount an increased systolic blood pressure response to exercise indicates an abnormal left ventricle. This is an indication to stop the test. In some cases the blood pressure may even drop on exercise, and this is indicative of a worse prognosis. Possible underlying causes may include coronary artery disease, valve disease or underlying cardiomyopathy.

Ventricular arrhythmias

In the majority of cases, ventricular arrhythmias alone are not specific to coronary artery disease. However, if accompanied by chest pain or ST depression, they are more specific. VT that occurs on exercise requires further investigation.

Ventricular rate

Failure to mount an increased heart rate may be the result of the patient being on beta-blockers or rate-limiting calcium-channel blockers. If the patient is not on any rate-limiting drugs, this is an abnormal response to exercise.

Echocardiography

Echocardiography is an extremely useful investigation, but its indications and limitations must be appreciated in order to obtain maximum benefit. It uses ultrasound to generate images that are viewed on a screen.

Advantages
- It displays real-time information.
- All machines are portable, so it is a useful quick bedside test.
- It provides good temporal resolution, so can image moving structures.
- It is a relatively cheap investigation.
- It can be used for patients with pacemakers (where MRI is contraindicated).

Disadvantages
- Some patients have poor echo 'windows' (e.g. obese individuals, and those with chronic lung disease or a history of previous cardiothoracic surgery). This makes clear images difficult to obtain.

- There is inter-observer variability.
- Images must be 'on axis' for accurate measurements to be made.

Indications

The British Society of Echocardiography has published recommended indications for requesting an echocardiogram. When requesting this investigation, try to adhere to these. The full list can be found at www.bsecho.org

Always check whether a recent echocardiogram has been performed (within the last 6 months), as there are few indications for a repeat study. Discuss the need with your local echocardiography department.

Important points when requesting an echocardiogram

- Document as much clinical information as possible on the request form. This will help the operator to answer the question that has been posed. If the patient has had a recent MI, state this (and which territory). If they have a valve replacement, state the date of surgery and the type of valve (if known), as normal values vary between different prosthetic valves. The results of the echocardiogram will be much more useful to the doctor and the patient if the technician has a specific clinical question to answer.
- If an 'urgent' echocardiogram is required, speak directly with the echo department rather than simply writing 'urgent' on the form. This will improve inter-departmental relations and benefit your patient.
- Do not simply request an echocardiogram because your senior has asked for it. If you are uncertain why it is being requested, ask your senior. If they do not know, it is unlikely that it needs to be done.
- Check heart rate and rhythm. It is difficult to obtain accurate measurements of LV function if a patient is in rapid AF.

Contrast echocardiography

Agitated saline or commercially available echo contrast agents can be injected intravenously at the time of echocardiography in order to obtain the following additional information:

- to improve endocardial border definition
- to assess for holes and shunts, particularly at inter-atrial level.

The decision to use contrast is usually made by the echocardiographer if the image quality is insufficient to answer the clinical question. They will often contact a member of the medical team to administer the contrast IV.

Stress echocardiography

The availability of this investigation varies widely between institutions. Either pharmacological stress or exercise can be used immediately before or during echocardiography. Drugs such as dobutamine and adenosine are commonly used.

Indications

1 Chest pain evaluation (non-diagnostic stress ECG, intermediate CAD likelihood):
   - resting ST/T-wave abnormalities
   - left bundle branch block
   - ventricular paced rhythm
   - left ventricular hypertrophy
   - digoxin treatment.
2 CAD diagnosis, risk stratification and therapy:
   - identification of lesions causing perfusion defects when planning for coronary intervention.
3 Risk stratification prior to non-cardiac surgery.
4 Assessment of intra-cavity dynamic gradients (e.g. HCM).
5 Assessment of valvular disease on exercise (e.g. aortic stenosis).

Important points

- Adrenergic-stimulating agents should be avoided in patients with unstable angina, hypokalaemia, uncontrolled hypertension (resting systolic blood pressure > 200 mmHg or diastolic blood pressure > 110 mmHg), uncontrolled congestive heart failure or uncontrolled dysrhythmias.
- Vasodilator agents should not be used in patients with second- or third-degree atrioventricular block (without permanent pacemakers), or in patients with chronic asthma or severe chronic obstructive lung disease.
- The use of quantitative 'ejection fraction' as a measure of left ventricular systolic function is being increasingly recognised by cardiologists as an imperfect tool with significant inter-observer variability and inaccuracy for a variety of reasons. Qualitative statements such as 'good', 'mild', 'moderate' or 'severe' impairment are becoming more routinely used, and are generally more useful.

Dyssynchrony echocardiography

Echocardiography can be used to determine intra- and interventricular dyssynchrony. This has a role in heart failure, particularly when cardiac resynchronisation therapy is being considered, or has been implanted and requires optimisation. For this reason, dyssynchrony studies will often only be available in centres with expertise in cardiac devices, and should be primarily requested by cardiologists or physicians with a particular interest in this area.

If the surface ECG has a narrow QRS complex (a measure of electrical synchrony), it is unlikely that there will be underlying mechanical dyssynchrony.

Trans-oesophageal echocardiography

This is an invasive investigation, and in most circumstances a standard trans-thoracic echocardiogram should have been performed prior to a TOE, as these are not without risk. Conscious sedation is often required, although some patients tolerate TOE remarkably well. As this is a semi-invasive procedure, written consent is required. Although serious complications are rare (0.2% of cases), patients should be informed of the following potential complications:

- discomfort and sore throat
- bleeding
- aspiration
- perforation
- arrhythmia
- hypoxia
- laryngospasm.

Patients must be nil by mouth for more than 4 hours before the procedure, and must not consume hot food or drinks afterwards until the local anaesthetic spray at the back of the throat has completely worn off, to avoid potentially serious burns and aspiration. Patients with dentures must remove them prior to undergoing TOE. The procedure is similar to an upper GI endoscopy, except that the probe is passed blindly into the oesophagus. The transducer probe then sits in the mid-oesophagus and sometimes in the stomach, to reduce interference from lung tissue. It uses ultrasound at a higher frequency (3.5–7 MHz) than TTE (2–4 MHz). These factors aid the generation of higher-resolution images than those obtained from TTE.

Indications
- Valve disease:
  - — mitral valve – a detailed assessment can be made of most pathology
  - — aortic regurgitation/adjunct to assess aortic stenosis (this is often better with TTE)
  - — prosthetic valve dysfunction.
- Bacterial endocarditis.
- Cardiac source of embolism, including PFO.
- Aortic pathology:
  - — dissection, rupture, aneurysm and atheroma.
- Prior to DCCV (to exclude left atrial appendage thrombus which cannot be seen on TTE).
- Cardiac masses.
- Pericardial disease and masses.
- Congenital heart disease.
- Intra-operative monitoring, particularly for cardiothoracic surgery.
- Assessment of haemodynamics in sedated patients on the ICU.
- Guiding interventional procedures (e.g. ASD closure, ablation, mitral clip).
- Poor transthoracic windows.

Tilt-table testing

This test aims to simulate reflex syncope triggered by prolonged standing. Blood pooling and a reduction in venous return are followed by an increase in vagal tone, often associated with hypotension and bradycardia. Several protocols exist involving pharmacological provocation with drugs such as isoproterenol and nitrates. This is essentially a test of autonomic function. Most studies are used to confirm clinical suspicion. If a firm diagnosis has been made, tilt-table testing does not usually add much additional information except in special circumstances (*see* Indications), and is not recommended for assessment of treatment. Patients must be fasted for 4 hours before the test and have an intravenous cannula *in situ*.

Indications (European Society of Cardiology guidelines 2009)
1 Single syncopal episode in a high-risk setting (e.g. physical injury, occupational implications) in the absence of organic heart disease, or in the presence of organic heart disease after cardiac causes of syncope have been excluded.
2 To demonstrate susceptibility to reflex syncope to the patient.

3   To discriminate between reflex syncope and OH syncope.
4   To differentiate syncope with jerking movements from epilepsy.
5   To evaluate recurrent unexplained falls.
6   To evaluate frequent syncope and psychiatric disease.

Isoproterenol tilt testing is contraindicated in patients with ischaemic heart disease.

Diagnostic criteria
- In patients without structural heart disease the induction of reflex hypotension/bradycardia:
    - with reproduction of syncope or progressive OH (with or without symptoms) is diagnostic of reflex syncope and OH, respectively
    - without reproduction of syncope may be diagnostic of reflex syncope.
- In patients with structural heart disease, arrhythmia or other cardiovascular causes of syncope should be excluded before positive tilt test results are considered to be diagnostic.
- Induction of LOC in the absence of hypotension and/or bradycardia should be considered diagnostic of psychogenic pseudosyncope.

Complications and contraindications
- Although tilt testing is safe, resuscitation facilities should be available during the procedure.
- Ventricular arrhythmias – very rare, but have been reported with isoproterenol use in ischaemic heart disease.
- Atrial fibrillation – usually self-limiting.
- Palpitations with isoproterenol.
- Headache with nitrate.
- Avoid these drugs in patients with LVOT obstruction or severe aortic stenosis.

Coronary angiography
Coronary angiography remains the gold standard investigation for anatomical evaluation of the coronary arteries. Access to this investigation varies between hospitals, which generally fall into one of four groups:
1   those with no access to a cardiac catheterisation laboratory
2   those with access to a catheter laboratory that only performs diagnostic angiography

3 those with a catheter laboratory equipped to perform 'simple' percutaneous intervention
4 cardiac centres capable of performing 'complex' percutaneous interventional procedures (including chronic coronary occlusions, left main stem
stenting and percutaneous valve replacement). These centres must have
on-site cardiothoracic surgical services.

Patients may be booked for:
- angiogram only
- angiogram plus the possibility of proceeding to PCI if necessary
- elective PCI.

Consent will be taken by the operator, and includes the risk of stroke, myocardial infarction, death, vascular injury, contrast nephropathy, bleeding
and arrhythmia. In general, for a diagnostic procedure the overall risk of
major complications is 0.1%, and for an interventional procedure it is 1%,
but individual cases may vary.

Before any procedure the following details must be obtained, and it is
often the responsibility of the junior doctor to ensure that this has been done.
- Recent FBC, U&E, clotting, and group and save.
- No low-molecular-weight heparin must be given within 12 hours of the
procedure.
- All patients who are having a radial procedure must have an
intravenous cannula sited, and Allen's test documented.
- All patients who are having an angiogram with the possibility of
proceeding to PCI, or who are having elective angioplasty, must have an
intravenous cannula sited.
- Details of any previous CABG or other cardiothoracic procedure,
including the location and type of graft(s) and/or valvular prosthesis.
- Details of any previous coronary intervention, including stent type, size and
location. There may be potential difficulties with access and/or anatomy.
- Details of any previous contrast reactions or allergy to shellfish
(increased risk of contrast reaction). This should prompt pre-treatment
with steroids and antihistamines (e.g. hydrocortisone 100 mg IV and
chlorpheniramine 10 mg IV).
- Details of any previous bleeding problems or peptic ulcer disease.
- Details of any known peripheral vascular disease. This must include
any known grafts (particularly Dacron grafts in the femoral region) or
any known abdominal aortic aneurysm (or repair). These are likely to
prompt a radial approach.

- Diabetic patients who are taking metformin must discontinue this drug 3–5 days before coronary angiography. It should not be re-started until the creatinine level has returned to baseline.

Special consideration

Patients with prosthetic heart valves who are on anticoagulation therapy must have this addressed prior to angiography. Management varies between institutions and between different types of valve, but the following general rules apply.
- Prosthetic mitral valves are more thrombogenic than aortic valves.
- Older prosthetic valves (e.g. ball in cage) are more thrombogenic than newer-generation (e.g. bi-leaflet) prosthetic valves.

As a result, a high-risk patient may be admitted before their procedure for discontinuation of oral anticoagulation, and implementation of intravenous heparin once the INR is below a certain threshold (there will be variation between different centres and operators, so it is advised that you discuss this with your seniors). Be aware that low-molecular-weight heparin does *not* have a licence for therapeutic anticoagulation for prosthetic valves, although it is sometimes used.

Contrast-induced nephropathy is more likely to occur with reduced baseline renal function. Estimated glomerular filtration rate is a much more accurate measure of this than serum creatinine levels. If impaired, pre-treatment with intravenous hydration (caution is needed in patients with severe heart failure and valvular heart disease) and N-acetyl cysteine is recommended (follow the local guidelines).

Contrast-induced nephropathy is not usually apparent until 3–5 days after the procedure. Patients with impaired baseline renal function who are being discharged before this time must have repeat renal function sent at a suitable time interval in order to identify any deterioration. These results must be followed up either by the hospital team or by the GP. If the GP is to follow them up, they must be informed of this!

The procedure

Coronary angiography is an invasive investigation that requires access to the arterial circulation, usually via either the femoral or radial arteries. Local anaesthetic is administered and a sheath is inserted using the Seldinger technique. Through this sheath a series of wires and plastic catheters can be passed and manoeuvred into coronary ostia.

Iodinated contrast medium is then injected through the catheters and fluoroscopy is used to obtain images. Images are acquired in different orthogonal planes to ensure that stenoses are not missed. Images of the left ventricle and aorta may also be taken. Once all of the diagnostic data have been collected, the sheaths are removed and haemostasis is achieved using either direct manual pressure or a vascular access occlusion device.

Other catheter laboratory procedures

- Right heart catheterisation is similar to left heart catheterisation, except that venous access (usually the femoral or jugular veins) is obtained rather than arterial access. This can be useful in the assessment of valvular heart disease, pulmonary arterial hypertension, intra-cardiac shunts, and to distinguish restrictive cardiomyopathy from pericardial constriction.
- Percutaneous valvular procedures.
- Percutaneous cardiac defect (e.g. PFO/ASD) closure.
- Endomyocardial biopsy.
- Invasive electrophysiology procedures.

Post-procedure complications to be aware of on the ward

The most common complication that you need to be aware of is bleeding at the access site. This is more of a problem with femoral procedures, as the site is 'hidden.' Beware of the shocked patient. Retroperitoneal haemorrhage is a potentially life-threatening condition and must be recognised early. It is usually a consequence of high puncture of the posterior wall of the common femoral artery. Suspect it if there are signs of shock and pain during an ipsilateral straight leg raise post procedure. The diagnosis is best made by CT, and treatment involves emergency surgery.

Pseudoaneurysm should be suspected if a bruit is heard over the femoral artery, with an expansile mass on palpation. The diagnosis is made by ultrasound scanning. Treatment may involve extended manual compression or may require injection of thrombin into the neck of the pseudoaneurysm. Both may be very painful, and appropriate analgesia must be prescribed.

Arrhythmias are usually self-limiting, but ventricular arrhythmias must be identified and promptly treated.

A rash typical of a drug reaction can occur as a result of contrast agents. These are often self-limiting, but may need treatment with chlorpheniramine and/or steroids. Serious anaphylactoid reactions are much less common, and are more likely to occur as an acute phenomenon on the catheter lab table than later on the ward.

Chest pain is a fairly common complaint in patients, particularly following stent implantation. This is often benign, but complications such as vessel dissection, thrombosis, spasm and perforation must be excluded. If possible, inform the operator that their patient has chest pain. Arrange an urgent ECG and compare it with the previous one. A trial of sublingual nitrate may be useful.

6

Primary and secondary prevention of cardiovascular disease

Primary versus secondary prevention

Cardiovascular disease accounts for a huge proportion of morbidity and mortality in the UK. We invest hundreds of millions of pounds in primary and secondary preventive measures each year, but still cardiovascular disease remains one of the most common causes of death in the UK.

The majority of primary prevention is carried out by general practitioners, while secondary prevention is by and large initiated by hospital practitioners and maintained by GPs.

* **Primary prevention.** This involves the identification of individuals at risk of developing cardiovascular disease, and treating them *before* the development of disease.
* **Secondary prevention.** Where disease has been established to any degree, secondary prevention aims to limit any progression of disease or its deterioration.

Risk factors

In an attempt to prevent cardiovascular disease at either the primary or secondary level, we need to consider risk factors. Some risk factors have more significance than others, but all can be divided into the categories of 'modifiable' and 'non-modifiable.'

TABLE 6.1 Modifiable and non-modifiable risk factors

MODIFIABLE RISK FACTORS	NON-MODIFIABLE RISK FACTORS
Smoking	Diabetes
Hypercholesterolaemia	Age
Hypertension	Family history/genetics
Sedentary lifestyle	Ethnicity
Obesity	

Although diabetes can be classified as a 'non-modifiable' risk factor, it is perhaps not quite so clear cut. Previous studies, such as the United Kingdom Prospective Diabetes Study (UKPDS), have clearly shown that the cardiovascular complications of diabetes can be significantly reduced by controlling other factors such as hypertension and glycaemic control. However, for the purposes of practical clinical knowledge one should probably continue to classify diabetes as a 'non-modifiable' risk factor.

Primary prevention

We would naturally presume that the majority of cardiovascular events occur in individuals within the so-called 'high risk' group. However, it is in fact those within the 'moderate-risk' group that suffer the majority of events, which is in part due to this being the largest patient group.

Data from the Framingham trials are used to calculate an individual's 10-year risk of developing cardiovascular disease. The charts can be found at the back of the *British National Formulary*, and are categorised into high, moderate and low risk of a cardiovascular event occurring within the next 10 years, where:

- high risk = 20% or higher chance of a cardiovascular event occurring in the next 10 years
- moderate risk = 10–19% chance of a cardiovascular event occurring in the next 10 years
- low risk = less than 10% chance of a cardiovascular event occurring in the next 10 years.

We use these data almost religiously, but it is important to consider some significant factors. The Framingham Study was conducted on a population from Framingham in Massachusetts, and is therefore of limited value for a diverse population. Furthermore, the study only covered individuals aged

30–62 years, and therefore may inaccurately predict cardiovascular events in patients outside this age range. Finally, the Framingham Study does not take into account family history, but genetics has an increasingly recognised role in predicting disease patterns and response to treatment.

Secondary prevention

After a primary cardiovascular event, strategies for prevention of future events must be implemented. In essence this will involve management of cardiac risk factors as well as 'having a healthy, balanced lifestyle.'

Areas to be addressed include the following:
- dietary modifications
- adherence to recommended alcohol intake
- physical exercise and optimisation of body weight
- smoking cessation
- cholesterol levels
- blood pressure
- diabetes (*see* UKPDS recommendations).

Dietary modifications
- A diet high in omega-3 fatty acids (7 g per week) is recommended. Omega-3-acid ethyl esters are licensed for secondary prevention after myocardial infarction (e.g. Omacor, which is prescribed at a dose of 1 g daily).
- A reduced intake of salt and saturated fats is advised.
- A Mediterranean-style diet is recommended.

Alcohol intake
- The recommended weekly allowance is 14 units for women and 21 units for men. This should not be exceeded.
- There is some evidence to suggest that red wine has beneficial cardiovascular effects due to the fact that it contains procyanidins and polyphenols (the French paradox).
- Some patients with extremely high levels of alcohol consumption may benefit from referral to a drugs and alcohol unit.
- Alcohol is of particular importance in heart failure, as it can be a cardiotoxin resulting in a dilated cardiomyopathy.

Physical exercise
- Regular cardiovascular exercise, such as swimming, running, walking

and cycling, is advised. Patients should avoid isometric exercise (e.g. heavy lifting) in the early months after a myocardial infarction.
- Exercising for 20–30 minutes per day, enough to induce slight breathlessness, is recommended.

Smoking cessation
- Patients must be encouraged to stop smoking. If they require help with this, they should be offered referral to a smoking cessation service.

Cholesterol
- Lowering cholesterol levels has beneficial effects on cardiovascular morbidity and mortality. There is no lower limit for cholesterol.
- The target for total cholesterol should be < 4 mmol/l, and the target for LDL-cholesterol should be < 2 mmol/l.

Blood pressure
- In general, the suggested treatment target is < 140/85 mmHg, and < 130/80 mmHg in high-risk patients. There is some evidence to suggest that diabetic patients with diabetic nephropathy should have a target of < 125/75 mmHg.

Diabetic patients
- Tight blood pressure control, glycaemic control, and reducing weight and cholesterol levels are important in this particularly vulnerable group of patients.
- Diabetic patients require a multi-disciplinary team approach to their care in order to minimise cardiovascular and other complications.

Further reading
Relevant NICE guideline (http://guidance.nice.org.uk):
- *MI: Secondary Prevention.* CG 48. May 2007.

7

Ischaemic heart disease

Epidemiology

Ischaemic heart disease is the most common cause of death in the UK. More than 1.4 million people have angina, and 275 000 people each year have a myocardial infarction.[1]

Mortality from IHD shows marked geographical variation within the UK, with higher death rates in Scotland compared with the south of England. Variation can also be found within the UK when comparing occupations, social class and ethnic groups.

Aetiology

It is important to risk-stratify patients by assessing their risk factors for ischaemic heart disease. As you would expect, the more risk factors an individual has, the higher is the probability that they will have significant IHD.

When evaluating risk factors, consider both those that are reversible and those that are irreversible (*see* Chapter 6). Many risk factors have been described, including 'stress', although definitive evidence for this is lacking.

Clinical presentation
- Chest pain.
- Radiation.
- Dyspnoea.
- Diaphoresis (excessive sweating).
- Nausea.
- Palpitations.
- Pre-syncope/syncope.

The way in which a patient presents, and their clinical state, will vary enormously. Some patients will appear relatively stable, while others may be extremely unwell, or in shock, requiring senior input from an early stage.

The following findings should alert you to the need to seek senior help early on:
- loss of cardiac output (put out an arrest call)
- impaired consciousness level in a previously well patient
- hypotensive patient despite fluid resuscitation
- new arrhythmias
- profoundly bradycardic patient (check whether they are on a beta-blocker)
- pain that is refractory to analgesia and GTN (the patient may require GTN infusion and/or a glycoprotein IIb/IIIa inhibitor)
- dynamic ECG changes
- STEMI.

Initial assessment must include heart rate, blood pressure, oxygen saturations and blood glucose, as well as examination of heart sounds, lung fields, and femoral and radial pulses. Be aware of other urgent differentials (e.g. aortic dissection, GI bleed) and acute complications (e.g. myocardial rupture) where you would want to avoid urgent thrombolytic or anticoagulant treatments.

Initial investigations
- **ECG.** Look for signs of ischaemia in a specific territory. Identify any conduction defects, as some of these may require rapid intervention.
- **FBC.** There may not be a primary cardiac problem, as anaemia of any cause can result in chest pain. A neutrophil leucocytosis may occur.
- **U&E.** Look specifically at the patient's renal function. A GFR of < 30 ml/min will require a 50% reduction in the dose of low-molecular-weight heparin.
- **Cardiac enzymes.** Check your local trust guidelines. Some trusts will check a troponin level at 12 hours, while others will check a baseline *and* a 6-hour or 12-hour troponin level.
- **Chest X-ray.** Look for evidence of heart failure and pulmonary oedema, which may complicate an acute cardiac event. It is also important to exclude other possible causes of chest pain, such as pneumonia and aortic dissection.

Investigations that are sometimes required

- **D-dimer.** This test should not be routine, but may be useful in the context of atypical chest pain, or to exclude a pulmonary embolism in certain circumstances.
- **ABG.** This is not necessary for all patients, but may be important in the acutely unwell patient for a variety of reasons.

Diagnostic investigations

ECG

This is a non-invasive and extremely valuable diagnostic aid. Ensure that you are familiar with the ECG indications for thrombolysis/primary PCI. The ECG may help you to identify the coronary artery that is likely to be responsible. Request serial ECGs in patients with chest pain. Repeat ECGs should be 15–20 minutes apart. Leave the electrode tabs in the same place to avoid variation in lead position.

TABLE 7.1 Infarct area with corresponding ECG and vascular territory

TERRITORY	CORRESPONDING ECG LEADS	CORONARY ARTERIAL SUPPLY
Anteroseptal	V1–V4	LAD
Inferior	II, III and aVF	RCA
Anterolateral	V4–V6, I and aVL	LAD or Cx
Lateral	I, aVL ± V5–V6	LCx
Posterior	Tall R-wave in V1–V2	Usually LCx, also RCA

Cardiac enzymes

Cardiac enzymes are an extremely useful adjunct to making a diagnosis of IHD, but must not be relied upon. The main enzymes are troponin I and troponin T, creatine phosphokinase (CPK), lactate dehydrogenase (LDH) and aspartate aminotransferase (AST). All of these enzymes rise and peak at different times, with varying half-lives. Troponin is the most commonly used marker of cardiac injury, and its activity is proportional to the size of infarction. Remember that other pathologies may also cause a rise in troponin activity. These include the following:

- renal failure
- pulmonary embolism
- severe sepsis
- prolonged tachycardia

- heart failure
- pancreatitis
- extreme physical exertion.

TABLE 7.2 Cardiac enzymes

MARKER	INITIAL RISE	PEAK	RETURN TO BASELINE
Myoglobin	1–4 hours	6–7 hours	24 hours
CPK	4–8 hours	18 hours	2–3 days
Troponin	3–12 hours	24 hours	3–10 days
LDH	10 hours	24–48 hours	14 days

The use of enzymes is important when distinguishing between the acute coronary syndromes. Both STEMI and NSTEMI can only be diagnosed when there is a significant increase in cardiac enzyme activity. You should bear in mind that troponin I is more sensitive than troponin T. Chest pain accompanied by ECG changes in the absence of a rise in cardiac enzyme activity should be termed angina (stable if brought on by stress, and unstable if present at rest).

Transthoracic echocardiogram

This may be a useful initial test in specialist centres, but is not routinely available in most centres as an initial investigation. It can aid the diagnosis of a variety of conditions acutely, such as torrential mitral regurgitation secondary to MI (as a result of chordal rupture).

Regional wall motion abnormalities are an important finding after MI. These are areas of the myocardium that have been either 'stunned' or rendered akinetic by the insult of ischaemia, and no longer contract in the correct manner. Some of this function may recover over time. The ejection fraction may be affected initially, but may also recover partially or completely over time. It is helpful for the echocardiographer if you write a brief history and what you are looking for (e.g. *42-year-old male with ST depression in leads II, III and aVF and troponin 3.27 on 17/08/09. ?RWMA and ejection fraction*).

Coronary angiography

This is the definitive investigation for patients with ischaemic heart disease. Coronary angiography should only be requested by a consultant or specialist registrar in cardiology. In the acute setting, patients who may benefit from primary PCI should be discussed with seniors as a medical emergency.

Consent is required for this investigation, and must only be sought by a consultant cardiologist or a cardiology specialist registrar.

Exercise ECG
Before this investigation is requested, ensure that there are no contraindications such as acute MI, myocarditis, severe aortic stenosis, adults with complete heart block, any recent pyrexial or 'flu-like' illness, unstable angina or uncontrolled hypertension. Ensure that your patient has reasonable mobility before requesting exercise testing. It is not uncommon for a patient who is not capable of walking further than 100 metres to be sent for exercise testing.

Cardiac CT
This is a 'triple rule-out' test which can diagnose coronary disease, pulmonary emboli and aortic dissection. This investigation is currently only available in specialist centres, although its use is very likely to become more widespread. The radiation dose is equivalent to that in coronary angiography, but it is non-invasive. As a general rule, cardiac CT is best performed in patients with regular heart rhythms. Images are of poorer quality in the presence of tachycardia. The test uses iodinated contrast medium, with regard to which the normal cautions and contraindications apply.

Perfusion imaging
This is usually done with nuclear medicine scanning, although some centres are using cardiac MRI. Pictures of the heart are taken at rest, and then after pharmacological stress. A regional difference implies a stenosis in the artery that is supplying that territory. If positive, this may prompt onward referral for coronary angiography with or without revascularisation.

Diagnosis of angina, NSTEMI and STEMI
Ischaemic heart disease is an umbrella term that encompasses angina, non-ST elevation myocardial infarction and ST-elevation myocardial infarction. The latter two (STEMI and NSTEMI) are known as acute coronary syndromes (ACS).

History
This is essential to making a diagnosis of IHD. Although chest pain is an important feature of IHD, do consider the atypical presentations such as neck pain, abdominal pain, or even no pain in a diabetic or elderly patient, who will often just complain of breathlessness.

ECG

The ECG can help to differentiate each stage of ischaemic heart disease, as summarised below.

Angina

- Usually normal between attacks.
- ST-segment depression and/or T-wave inversion in a vascular territory can be provoked by stress (e.g. on treadmill testing, under anaesthesia, or in the context of anaemia).

NSTEMI

- May show evidence of previous ischaemic cardiac events.
- ST-segment depression and/or T-wave inversion in a vascular territory.
- Planar or down-sloping ST-segment depression is a better predictor of ischaemia than T-wave inversion.

STEMI

- ST elevation of ≥ 1 mm in two or more limb leads.
- ST elevation of ≥ 2 mm in two or more contiguous chest leads.
- Remember that the diagnostic criteria for thrombolysis of a STEMI also encompass new or presumed new LBBB.

There is no reason why any patient who attends hospital (Accident and Emergency or Medical Admissions Unit) should not have an ECG done. It is a cheap, non-invasive investigation which has many important diagnostic qualities. It is good practice to give any patient with a resting abnormal ECG a copy to take with them which can be used for comparison at future presentations to hospital.

Risk stratification

TIMI scoring

This must not be confused with thrombolysis in myocardial infarction (TIMI) flow grade, which is an angiographic measurement. TIMI scoring is a convenient method of determining an individual's 14-day risk of experiencing a cardiac event after presentation with either UA or NSTEMI. It is therefore useful when risk-stratifying individuals, particularly when determining onward referrals for further investigations.

TABLE 7.3 TIMI risk assessment scoring system

HISTORY	POINTS
Age ≥ 65 years	1
≥ 3 CAD risk factors (FHx, HTN, raised cholesterol, DM, active smoker)	1
Known CAD (stenosis ≥ 50%)	1
ASA use in past 7 days	1
Presentation	
Recent (≤ 24 hours) severe angina	1
Cardiac markers	1
ST deviation ≥ 0.5 mm	1

Risk score = total points (0–7)

TABLE 7.4 Percentage risk of cardiac event at day 14

RISK OF CARDIAC EVENTS (%) BY 14 DAYS IN TIMI 11B*		
RISK SCORE	DEATH OR MI	DEATH, MI OR URGENT REVASCULARISATION
0/1	3	5
2	3	8
3	5	13
4	7	20
5	12	26
6/7	19	41

* Entry criteria: UA or NSTEMI defined as ischaemic pain at rest within the past 24 hours, with evidence of CAD (ST segment deviation or positive marker).

Reproduced from Antman *et al.* 2000 *JAMA.* **284**: 835–42.

Management

Medical management

Management of patients with IHD should be considered in terms of:

1 primary prevention
2 secondary prevention
3 emergency management.

Primary prevention involves risk-stratifying patients with regard to their 10-year cardiovascular risk and working with them to modify any risk factors if they have not experienced any cardiac events to date. Secondary prevention

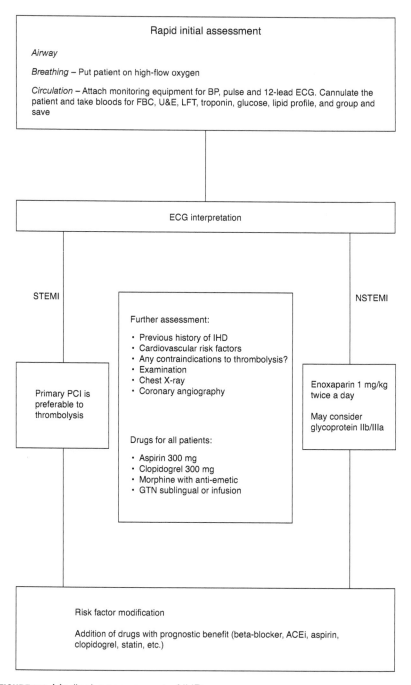

FIGURE 7.1 Medical management of IHD.

involves the application of the same principles to those who have already had a myocardial infarction (for further details, *see* Chapter 6).

Emergency management of patients with acute coronary syndromes necessitates prompt treatment, as 'time is muscle.'

Surgical management

Surgical treatment is usually elective in the context of IHD. Occasionally there may be an indication for urgent surgical management, as in the following:

- torrential MR secondary to papillary muscle rupture from acute MI
- type A aortic dissection.

Surgical management of IHD is more commonly decided upon after the acute event has passed and the patient has undergone coronary angiography. Traditionally a patient with triple-vessel disease, left main stem disease, or diffuse disease not amenable to PCI should be considered for CABG surgery. Increasingly 'complex' PCI is being performed in these patient groups at specialist centres.

Daily monitoring/investigations

1 Close observation of vital signs.
2 If a patient has been diagnosed with an MI but has not yet undergone angiography, they should remain on ECG telemetry to observe for arrhythmias.
3 Daily examination, looking specifically for any signs of heart failure, new cardiac murmurs and further episodes of chest pain.
4 Daily ECG, looking for conduction abnormalities, Q-waves or further ischaemic events.
5 Repeat cardiac enzymes the following day to ensure that enzyme activity levels are falling.

Any further episodes of pain should be taken seriously, and would warrant repeating all of the above steps.

Important tips

Cardiology

Discuss the case with a cardiologist in order to obtain any specialist advice and guidance on appropriate investigations for each patient. It is also important to establish with cardiology what kind of follow-up is appropriate. After the acute event, it is useful to request investigations such as a transthoracic echo before a referral to cardiology is made.

You should not assume that a patient with ECG changes and no rise in troponin levels can merely go home. After risk stratification, it may be apparent that the patient requires further investigation as described above.

Cannulae
Intravenous cannulae are a common source of infection in hospitals. Ensure that you change the cannula every 3 days, and inspect the cannula sites daily for early signs of local infection. Write the date of insertion on the cannula dressing, and record this in the notes to avoid confusion.

Previous records
Review the patient's case notes, particularly for details of previous cardiac investigations such as cardiac catheterisation, echocardiograms, exercise tolerance testing, myocardial perfusion scans, etc.

Information to have to hand for ward rounds
1 Up-to-date bloods, including FBC, U&E, LFT, CRP, cardiac enzymes, fasting cholesterol and fasting glucose.
2 Serial ECGs from admission. Label them in order of time, with documentation of pain scores and any medications given.
3 Notification of any arrhythmias while the patient was on telemetry. Print these off for the consultant to review.
4 The results of the most recent echocardiogram or the date when echo is booked.
5 Any previous cardiac investigation results (echocardiogram, angiogram, myocardial perfusion scan, dobutamine stress echocardiography, exercise tolerance test, 24-hour tape, etc.).
6 Current medication regimen (aspirin, clopidogrel, statin, ACEi, beta-blocker, low-molecular-weight heparin, glycoprotein IIb/IIIa, etc.). If a patient is not on a prognostically beneficial medication, the reason for this must be known.
7 Observation chart for temperature and haemodynamic status.

Reference

1   www.dh.gov.uk/en/Healthcare/NationalServiceFrameworks/Coronaryheart disease/index.htm

Further reading

Relevant NICE guidelines (http://guidance.nice.org.uk):

- *Chest Pain of Recent Onset.* CG 95. March 2010.
- *Unstable Angina and NSTEMI.* CG 94. March 2010.

8

Heart failure

Heart failure is a clinical syndrome in which the heart is unable to supply sufficient blood flow to meet demands. It is possible to have heart failure without clinical evidence of fluid accumulation.

Epidemiology

As with many chronic disease processes, the prevalence of heart failure increases with age. Approximately 1% of men and women under the age of 65 years have heart failure. This figure rises dramatically to 12–22% in men and women aged 85 years or over. As a result, heart failure is a significant burden on the healthcare system.

Aetiology

There are many causes of heart failure, and it is important to differentiate between them in order to ensure correct treatment and follow-up. You must always remember the context in which the patient presents – a 90-year-old patient with breathlessness will probably not need the full battery of investigations that would be required for a 40-year-old.

Heart failure may be an acute or chronic phenomenon and may affect the left or right ventricle, or both. Diastolic heart failure refers to the heart's inability to relax, often as a result of reduced ventricular compliance. It is common in amyloidosis, hypertension and cardiomyopathy where the heart muscle is 'stiff.'

Important causes of heart failure include the following:
- coronary ischaemia
- hypertension
- valvular causes
- myocarditis and post-viral cardiomyopathy

- idiopathic dilated cardiomyopathy
- familial causes
- infiltrative (amyloid, sarcoid, iron overload)
- chemotherapy
- radiotherapy
- postpartum
- primary heart muscle disease
- alcohol
- endocrine (particularly thyroid)
- tachyarrhythmia
- infections (Chagas disease)
- nutritional (beriberi).

Clinical presentation

History

Points to document in the clerking include the following:

- Symptoms of breathlessness:
  — duration
  — orthopnoea (ask how many pillows the patient uses when sleeping)
  — paroxysmal nocturnal dyspnoea.
- Exercise tolerance – quantify in terms of distance or time:
  — on the flat
  — on inclines or stairs.
- Peripheral oedema.
- Associated chest pain, palpitations, pre-syncope or syncope.
- Factors in the history that may give a clue to the underlying aetiology:
  — history of alcohol intake
  — history of hypertension
  — previous infarcts and/or risk factors for coronary artery disease
  — previous rheumatic heart disease
  — chemotherapy
  — thyroid status
  — recent infection
  — family history of heart failure.

Examination

There are several important points to note in the examination:

- Pulse – rhythm and rate are both important. Patients with AF commonly have a period of poor rate control (for a number of reasons), which results in the decompensation of their heart failure. In some cases it is particularly important to avoid drugs like beta-blockers, which may worsen an acute episode of heart failure.

- Jugular venous pressure is likely to be elevated. Bear in mind that some patients with biventricular failure will have tricuspid regurgitation, which will produce large 'v' waves in the JVP.
- Stigmata of chronic liver disease and hepatomegaly as a result of hepatic congestion.
- Mitral facies.
- Signs of thyroid disease.
- Blood pressure – patients with known heart failure often have a low blood pressure due to the intrinsic pump dysfunction, and the sheer number of pharmacological agents that they are taking (ACEi, beta-blocker, diuretics, nitrates, spironolactone, etc.).
- Heart sounds and murmurs – gallop rhythm, third heart sound.
- Oxygen saturation.
- Rales.
- Pitting peripheral oedema (remember that non-pitting oedema is common and may not be attributable to fluid overload from heart failure).

Initial investigations

- **ECG.** An entirely normal ECG makes heart failure unlikely. Often there will be voltage criteria for LVH, with or without evidence of left ventricular strain. There may be evidence of ventricular dyssynchrony which is demonstrated by prolonged QRS duration. Voltage size may be very small. Q waves may indicate previous MI. Look carefully as the ECG can give clues to the underlying aetiology.
- **Chest X-ray.** Look specifically for pleural effusions, fluid in the horizontal fissure, Kerley B lines (interstitial oedema), alveolar oedema ('bat's wings'), cardiomegaly and upper lobe blood diversion (*see* Figure 8.1).
- **FBC.** Symptoms of heart failure are likely to be more severe if the patient is anaemic. Anaemia may also precipitate heart failure. Haematinics and thyroid function tests should be sent if the patient is found to be anaemic.
- **U&E.** Patients with heart failure often require diuretics, which may impair renal function and also result in electrolyte imbalances. A baseline level should be ascertained prior to treatment, with regular

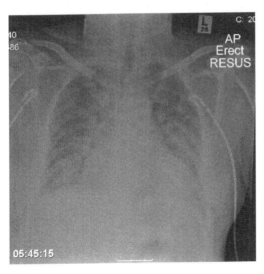

FIGURE 8.1 Plain film chest radiograph demonstrating features of acute heart failure.

monitoring. This is especially important with furosemide infusions and metolazone.

- **LFT.** Right heart failure and congestive cardiac failure can cause hepatic congestion with derangement of liver enzymes. Patients with worsening LFT or tender hepatomegaly should have a liver ultrasound examination to exclude gallbladder obstruction and evaluate the liver texture.
- **Brain natriuretic peptide (BNP).** This is a useful diagnostic adjunct in heart failure. However, it is not universally available. A concentration of > 400 pg/ml can predict heart failure with 90% sensitivity. It has a high negative predictive value, so is also useful for excluding heart failure as a diagnosis. Levels will be much higher in patients with chronic renal failure.
- **Thyroid function.** Hypothyroidism is a relatively uncommon cause of heart failure, but should be checked routinely, as this is a reversible cause.
- **Glucose.**
- In selected patients you may also wish to check the following:
  — ferritin (to screen for haemochromatosis)
  — immunoglobulins and serum protein electrophoresis (to screen for myeloma if you suspect amyloid heart disease)

   — viral titres (often taken if myocarditis is suspected, but seldom of any practical benefit).

- **Transthoracic echocardiogram** (*see* Chapter 7). When faced with a formal echocardiogram report, the various figures can seem quite confusing. The important features to note include the following:
  - left ventricular cavity size (small, normal or enlarged)
  - left ventricular wall thickness (note whether there is evidence of hypertrophy, and if so, whether this is concentric, which occurs in long-standing systemic hypertension; asymmetric hypertrophy of the septum occurs in hypertrophic cardiomyopathy)
  - any right ventricular involvement
  - the presence of pericardial and pleural fluid
  - calculate the left ventricular ejection fraction
  - any regional wall motion abnormalities, which may suggest previous myocardial infarction in that territory
  - significant valvular abnormality.

Further investigations

Cardiac MRI

This can be a useful investigation for determining the underlying aetiology of heart failure, but it is a specialised test and should not be requested without consultation with the cardiology team. Ensure that your patient does not have a pacemaker, as this will generally preclude MRI (although there are now some MRI-compatible devices available).

Holter monitoring

If chronic tachyarrhythmia (e.g. atrial fibrillation) is present, this can be a useful investigation for evaluating arrhythmic burden and rate profile.

Cardiopulmonary exercise testing

This provides an objective measurement of the patient's functional capacity. It is useful to predict prognosis and is also used in selecting patients for heart transplant. A six minute walk test is another useful way to objectively measure exercise capacity.

Pulmonary function testing

Pulmonary disease may coexist with heart failure. Basic spirometry, transfer factor and flow-volume loops can help to discriminate the cause of breathlessness.

Coronary angiogram

This will rule out significant coronary artery disease. Remember that if an artery is blocked the myocardium may be non-functioning. If this is the case, evidence of hibernation or viability should be sought prior to revascularisation, either by nuclear imaging, stress echocardiography or CMR. There is little evidence that asymptomatic patients should be screened for coronary disease.

Diagnostic criteria

The diagnosis of heart failure is made on the basis of a combination of clinical history and examination with supporting investigations. Patients should be classified in terms of a functional class, according to their symptoms. The most commonly used system is that of the New York Heart Association:

- Class I – patients have no limitation of their activity, and experience no symptoms from ordinary activities.
- Class II – patients have slight, mild limitation of their activity, and are comfortable when at rest or with mild exertion.
- Class III – patients have marked limitation of their activity, and are comfortable only at rest.
- Class IV – patients should be at complete rest, confined to bed or a chair; any physical activity brings on discomfort, and symptoms occur at rest.

Management

Medical management

Treatment of CCF should broadly be categorised as acute management or more chronic management, although general principles apply to both. More emphasis is placed on acute management here for the hospital junior doctor.

Management of acute pulmonary oedema

The patient who presents with acute pulmonary oedema can be a frightening prospect for the junior doctor, but can be one of the most satisfying cases to treat because there is often a dramatic clinical turnaround.

Remember ALS initially, and work in accordance with the ABC principles of acute medicine. Once the diagnosis has been confirmed, the following are necessary:

- oxygen to keep SpO_2 above 90%
- intravascular access

- urinary catheterisation with strict fluid balance monitoring, including admission and daily body weights
- a central venous line is often preferable, but if difficult should not delay treatment. Remember that these patients do not like lying flat, and it is therefore advised that they should be managed at an angle of 45–90°.

Identify and treat the underlying cause. Note that if it is secondary to acute coronary ischaemia, pulmonary oedema must be treated prior to invasive coronary procedures, as the patient must be able to lie flat to tolerate this. Drugs such as aspirin and clopidogrel are usually safe, but if imminent coronary angiography is being considered, low-molecular-weight heparin should be avoided.

Furosemide 40 mg IV can be repeated as necessary (onset of action is within approximately 6 minutes). It can also be given as an infusion if necessary (e.g. 5–10 mg/hour). It is preferable to give IV drugs in acute heart failure, as there is often gut oedema that limits absorption. Intravenous nitrates such as GTN (50 mg in 50 ml of normal saline infused at a rate of 2–10 ml/hour) often result in a dramatic improvement in the patient's clinical condition. Titrate upwards as necessary, keeping the systolic blood pressure above 100 mmHg.

If the patient remains hypoxic, continuous positive airway pressure (CPAP) ventilation should be considered. This will often need to be arranged via the CCU or ICU. It involves the use of a tight-fitting face mask through which oxygen is delivered with a PEEP of 5–10 cmH$_2$O. This helps to improve alveolar ventilation, and also reduces preload, which in turn reduces myocardial workload.

In cases of haemodynamic compromise, consider positive inotropic support. This should be given via a central vein by someone who is familiar with its use. You must therefore arrange this with your seniors. A discussion of individual regimens is beyond the scope of this book. It must be remembered that none of the drugs are perfect, as they will increase blood pressure and heart rate at the expense of increasing myocardial oxygen demand.

Low-dose inotropic drugs such as dopamine have been successfully used as a stabilising measure in CCF patients to support their blood pressure, allowing further off-loading with diuretic medication. This should always be carried out under specialist supervision.

Patients in cardiogenic shock, following an MI, may have an intra-aortic balloon pump (IABP) inserted in the cardiac catherisation laboratory. This balloon device sits in the descending aorta, where it is rapidly inflated and then deflates in time with the cardiac cycle. This reduces afterload and augments coronary filling in diastole. This is a highly specialised level of management, and is well beyond the scope of this book.

On occasion, intubation and mechanical ventilation in the ICU may have to be considered.

Pulmonary oedema that is unresponsive to medical therapy is an indication for emergency haemodialysis, and if needed this should be discussed with local intensive care or renal services. However, profound hypotension may preclude this.

Exceptions in acute pulmonary oedema

- Right ventricular infarction, which can be a complication of right coronary artery occlusion, and presents with hypotension, elevated JVP and clear lung fields. Right-sided ECG may help to make the diagnosis. These patients often require large volumes of fluid intravenously to maintain a satisfactory blood pressure. Invasive haemodynamic monitoring in an HDU or ICU setting together with central venous pressure with or without pulmonary arterial invasive pressure monitoring is often required. Vasodilators should be avoided if possible.
- Ventricular septal defect/free wall rupture has a grave prognosis even with prompt surgical intervention.
- Papillary muscle rupture should be suspected in cases that show clinical signs of mitral regurgitation, or sudden decompensation with a hyperdynamic circulation. The diagnosis is made by echocardiography, and treatment consists of urgent surgical intervention.
- Ischaemic mitral regurgitation is a phenomenon that is contributed to by left ventricular dysfunction. Initial treatment is of the underlying cause. A discussion of advanced interventional treatments is beyond the scope of this book.
- HCM with LVOT obstruction is complex. Paradoxically, vasodilation will make these patients worse, and treatment is with agents such as phenylephrine, which is a vasoconstrictor. These increase afterload but reduce the degree of LVOTO.
- Patients with severe decompensated valvular heart disease should be considered for emergency surgery in conjunction with local cardiologists and/or cardiothoracic surgeons. Remember that if a patient with known aortic stenosis is admitted with pulmonary oedema, *vasodilation can be fatal.* Treat the patient with diuretics and oxygen, and discuss them with your regional cardiac centre as a matter of urgency.

General measures

- Patients should be encouraged to monitor their weight in order to detect signs of fluid overload. If an obvious precipitant is found (e.g. thyroid disease, alcohol), this should be treated or withdrawn in conjunction with standard heart failure therapy.
- Patients should be put on fluid restriction (typically 1.5 litres per day).

Diet and alcohol

Patients should be encouraged to eat a low-salt diet to help to prevent worsening fluid retention. Alcohol consumption should be minimised, or stopped completely if implicated in the aetiology.

Pharmacological interventions

The treatment options are obviously related to the underlying cause, although there are general pharmacological therapies that apply to most heart failure treatments. Nephrotoxic drugs, particularly NSAIDs, should be withheld and alternatives sought. Try not to stop drugs in patients who are already established on heart failure therapy. Abrupt withdrawal of ACEi can in fact make the acute episode worse. It may be necessary to reduce the doses, but be guided by the patient's blood pressure and renal function.

Drugs for symptoms

- Diuretics. These drugs reduce the symptoms of fluid overload. The most commonly used are loop diuretics such as furosemide. In mild heart failure these can be given orally, but they may need to be administered intravenously in hospital. Some cardiologists also use bumetanide in the latter setting. Bumetanide 1 mg is roughly equivalent to furosemide 40 mg, but is better absorbed. Potent thiazide diuretics such as metolazone are used to treat refractory cases, but should only be prescribed on senior advice, due to the associated risk of nephrotoxicity.
- Potassium-sparing diuretics have less of a role, but can be considered in patients with hypokalaemia that persists despite ACEi and diuretics. Remember that oral potassium supplements are unpleasant tasting so compliance will be reduced.
- Patients in hospital should have daily renal function tests, especially if they require intravenous diuretics. Some cardiologists advocate temporary cessation of other nephrotoxic drugs (even prognostic drugs) during aggressive fluid off-loading, in order to avoid excessive nephrotoxicity.

- Digoxin. This is a weak positive inotrope that has been shown to reduce hospitalisations for heart failure even in patients with sinus rhythm (in the DIG trial), and it is indicated for patients with moderate heart failure. It is also useful for controlling rate in supraventricular arrhythmia in CCF patients. Digoxin can accumulate, particularly in patients with renal failure and in the elderly, so remember to check levels if this is suspected. The trough level should be 0.5–1.0 ng/ml.

Drugs for prognosis

- Angiotensin-converting-enzyme inhibitors (ACEi) and angiotensin-2-receptor blockers (A2RBs). There are various ACEi and A2RBs on the market, and opinion varies as to their relative superiority. There is good evidence that all of them improve morbidity and mortality. They are the first class of prognostic drug that should be started in CHF, and you should aim to establish the patient on the maximum tolerated dose.
- Beta-blockers. There is evidence that certain beta-blockers reduce mortality in heart failure. Currently only carvedilol, bisoprolol and metoprolol are approved by NICE. Beta-blockers should be avoided in acute pulmonary oedema. If a patient is on a non-cardioselective beta-blocker, and has evidence of heart failure, this should be switched to one of the drugs mentioned above.

TABLE 8.1 Dosing regimen of NICE approved beta-blockers

DRUG	FIRST DOSE	INCREMENTS	TARGET DOSE
Carvedilol	3.125 mg twice a day	6.25, 12.5, 25, 50	50 mg daily in divided doses
Bisoprolol	1.25 mg once daily	2.5, 3.75, 5, 7.5, 10	10 mg daily
Metoprolol	12.5 mg twice a day	25, 50, 100	100 mg daily in divided doses

Record an ECG before initiating beta-blocker therapy. Monitor the patient for bradycardia, blood pressure and clinical response. If the heart rate drops below 50 beats/min, consider halving the dose. If the patient is symptomatic, stop the drug. There is no need to reduce the dose for PR interval prolongation, but do monitor for signs of this. Note that beta-blockers should not be withdrawn abruptly, due to the risk of rebound symptoms. During acute deteriorations, there is evidence to suggest that reducing the dose is of greater prognostic benefit than cessation of the drug followed by re-initiation.

- Spironolactone. The aldosterone antagonist spironolactone has a significant (30%) mortality benefit in patients with NYHA class III or IV heart failure (demonstrated by the RALES study). The typical dose is 12.5–25 mg, with a maximum dose of 50 mg. Monitor for associated hyperkalaemia. If the K^+ concentration exceeds 6 mmol/l, stop the drug. If it is in the range 5.5–5.9 mmol/l, the drug can be continued at half the dose.

- Eplerenone is a newer aldosterone antagonist for which there is evidence of effectiveness in heart failure complicating myocardial infarction. Although it has fewer side-effects, it is significantly more expensive than spironolactone, and may not be included in the hospital formulary.
- Vasodilators. These drugs are generally not helpful in CCF. The combination of dinitrate and hydralazine has a mortality benefit in black patients with CCF, although the reason for this is unclear.
- Antiplatelet agents (e.g. aspirin, clopidogrel) are recommended only for patients with ischaemic cardiomyopathy.
- Anticoagulants. Patients with CCF and atrial fibrillation/flutter should be formally anticoagulated so long as there is no compelling contraindication. Patients with dilated ventricles or atria, or those with a left ventricular aneurysm or intracardiac thrombus, should also be considered for anticoagulation.

Renal function and cardiac drugs

Some deterioration in renal function is common with the administration of diuretics and ACEi in patients with CCF. It is the junior doctor's responsibility to ensure that bloods are taken at baseline and with changes in therapy, or daily if the patient is on intravenous therapy. An increase in creatinine levels to 50% above baseline or 200 µmol/l, whichever is the smaller, is acceptable so long as it is monitored and subsequent doses are withheld if this threshold is exceeded. An increase in K^+ concentration to ≤ 5.9 mmol/l is acceptable. Withhold non-essential nephrotoxic drugs and vasodilators during a period of worsening renal function. Deterioration above the thresholds stated should prompt discontinuation of drugs and consultation with the registrar or consultant.

Miscellaneous

- Gout is common in CCF, and should be treated with colchicine in the acute phase, followed by preventive therapy with allopurinol. Avoid NSAIDs and steroids.
- Anaemia is very common in CCF, and is often multifactorial in nature. Iron deficiency should be looked for and treated. There is growing evidence for the use of EPO in heart failure.

- Tricyclic antidepressants should be avoided as they have the potential to cause arrhythmias.

Device therapy
The NICE guidelines recommend cardiac resynchronisation therapy with a pacing device (CRT-P) as a treatment option for patients with heart failure who fulfil all of the following criteria:
- They are currently experiencing or have recently experienced NYHA class III or IV symptoms.
- They are in sinus rhythm *either* with a QRS duration of 150 ms or longer estimated by standard ECG, *or* with a QRS duration of 120–149 ms estimated by ECG *and* mechanical dyssynchrony that is confirmed by echocardiography.
- They have a left ventricular ejection fraction of 35% or less.
- They are receiving optimal pharmacological therapy.

Cardiac resynchronisation therapy with a defibrillator device (CRT-D) may be considered for patients who fulfil the criteria for implantation of a CRT-P device as well as the criteria for use of an ICD device. ICDs are recommended for patients in the following categories:
- 'Secondary prevention' – that is, patients who present (in the absence of a treatable cause) with one of the following:
  — survival of a cardiac arrest due to either ventricular tachycardia (VT) or ventricular fibrillation (VF)
  — spontaneous sustained VT that is causing syncope or significant haemodynamic compromise
  — sustained VT without syncope or cardiac arrest, and an associated reduction in ejection fraction (LVEF of less than 35%) (no worse than class III of the NYHA functional classification of heart failure).
- 'Primary prevention' – that is, patients who have:
  — a history of previous (more than 4 weeks ago) myocardial infarction (MI) and *either* left ventricular dysfunction with an LVEF of less than 35% (no worse than class III of the NYHA functional classification of heart failure) *and* non-sustained VT on Holter (24-hour ECG) monitoring *and* inducible VT on electrophysiological testing, *or* left ventricular dysfunction with an LVEF of less than 30% (no worse than class III of the NYHA functional classification of heart failure) *and* QRS duration equal to or more than 120 milliseconds

— a familial cardiac condition with a high risk of sudden death, including long QT syndrome, hypertrophic cardiomyopathy, Brugada syndrome *or* arrhythmogenic right ventricular dysplasia (ARVD), *or* have undergone surgical repair of congenital heart disease.

The aim of CRT (also known as biventricular pacing) is to improve the heart's pumping efficiency by resynchronising the pumping action of the chambers. The chambers must therefore first be demonstrated to be dyssynchronous.

CRT involves the transvenous implantation into the heart of three leads which are connected to a pulse generator. Leads are placed in the right atrium and the right ventricle, and a third lead (the left ventricular lead) is usually placed via the coronary sinus. The coronary sinus runs posteriorly in the atrio-ventricular groove, with branches adjacent to the left ventricle which can then be paced across the epicardium. CRT-P devices allow both regulation of atrioventricular delay and restoration of synchronous contraction by pacing the right atrium and both ventricles. A cardioverter defibrillator function can be included with the pulse generator to defibrillate the heart in the event that a malignant ventricular arrhythmia is detected, and in this case the device is known as a CRT-D device.

Surgical management
Mechanical ventricular assist devices
The junior doctor should be aware that such devices exist, but would not be expected to understand their role and operation. They may be used as a bridge to transplant (so-called 'destination therapy') to support a patient's circulation until such time as a donor becomes available.

Transplant
Cardiac transplantation is the final option for suitable patients who have failed to respond to conventional therapy as described above. The availability of donors limits this as an option for the majority of heart failure patients. Transplantation is also associated with the need for lifelong immunosuppression and thus an increased risk of cancers.

Daily monitoring/investigations
1 Close observation of vital signs and daily weights.
2 Daily examination, looking specifically for any signs of heart failure.
3 Daily bloods. U&E and magnesium levels should be closely monitored in

patients who are on high doses of diuretics. This is especially important for those on furosemide infusions.

4   Once-daily lying/standing blood pressure measurements will give you a guide as to when the patient is off-loaded, and becoming slightly hypovolaemic.

Important tips
Diuretic dosing
- Furosemide: starting dose 20–40 mg, titrate up to achieve dry weight, maximum dose 400 mg (in practice, doses above 80 mg should be discussed with seniors).
- Bumetanide: starting dose 0.5–1 mg, titrate up to achieve dry weight, maximum dose 10 mg.
- Metolazone: starting dose 2.5 mg, maximum dose 10 mg. It is often given on alternate days.
- Consider dosing every other day or weekly to avoid nephrotoxicity.

Starting an ACEi
Explain to the patient that the first few doses may be associated with symptomatic hypotension, and tell them not to be alarmed by this. Consider nocturnal dosing at first to minimise the impact. Start at a low dose and titrate up. This can be done more quickly as an inpatient, but this should not be the sole reason for prolonging the patient's hospital stay. Monitor renal function and discontinue the drug if there is significant deterioration. This should then prompt further investigation with renal ultrasound and renal artery Doppler or MRI. Warn the patient about side-effects such as dry cough, and seek alternatives should this develop.

Beta-blockers
Beta-blockers are often not prescribed for patients with heart failure on the grounds that they have 'asthma' or airways disease. However, so long as there is not a significant reversible defect on pulmonary function testing, most patients tolerate these drugs well. Metoprolol is a short-acting cardioselective drug, so may be an appropriate trial in the beta-blocker-naive patient.

Heart failure teams
Many hospitals have dedicated heart failure teams with specialist nurses, and close links with community teams. They have been shown to have a positive effect on CHF patients through a combination of correct drug therapy,

consideration of aetiology, education and referral for rehabilitation. Patients should be discussed with the heart failure nurse on discharge with regard to continuing care in the community.

The previously stable patient

When a previously stable CCF patient presents to hospital, consider the reasons *why* this may have happened and document them accordingly:

- inappropriate reduction in therapy
- poor compliance with therapy
- new inappropriate therapy (e.g. negatively inotropic drugs such as calcium-channel blockers, NSAIDS which promote salt and water retention)
- arrhythmia
- myocardial ischaemia or infarction
- infection
- anaemia
- alcohol
- thromboembolism.

Daily weights

It seems to be particularly difficult to document this observation reliably. To help to prompt nursing staff, write 'daily weight' on the observation chart or even as a prescription on the drug chart at 7 am every morning. Patients must be weighed daily, and on the same set of scales. If a weight has varied dramatically over a short period of time, interpret this with caution and seek an alternative explanation (e.g. the use of different scales).

Previous records

Review the patient's case notes, particularly for details of previous echocardiograms, CMR, coronary angiography, MPS, etc. Look back through their previous medication regimens, and at the progression of their disease. Have recent clinic letters available.

Information to have to hand for ward rounds

1 Up-to-date bloods, including FBC, U&E, LFT and BNP.
2 ECG from the current admission. It is important to look specifically at the QRS duration for evidence of dyssynchrony (wide QRS).
3 The results of the most recent echocardiogram, or the date when an echo is booked.

4   Results of all previous cardiac investigations.
5   Drug regimen on admission as well as current drug regimen.
6   Admission weight, dry weight and daily weight chart.
7   Observation chart for temperature and haemodynamic status.

9

Atrial fibrillation and flutter

Epidemiology

Atrial fibrillation

Atrial fibrillation (AF) is a very common arrhythmia with a prevalence of 0.5–1% in the general population. The incidence increases with age, and approximately 20% of individuals aged 80 years will have AF. Atrial transport contributes up to 20% of cardiac output. In AF, organised atrial contraction is lost and replaced by chaotic atrial electrical activity.

Atrial flutter

Very little is known about the epidemiology of atrial flutter. It is certainly much less common than AF. However, atrial flutter remains one of the more common causes of supraventricular arrhythmia.

Aetiology

There are several causes which must be assessed for in the patient with AF.

Common causes

- Ischaemic heart disease.
- Valvular heart disease.
- Hypertension.
- Heart muscle disease (e.g. HCM).
- CCF.

Potentially reversible causes

- Post-operative.
- Related to infection (often chest or systemic infection).

- Thyroid disease.
- Myocarditis/pericarditis.
- Alcohol or other stimulants (e.g. caffeine).
- Pulmonary embolism.

Rare causes
- GUCH.
- Cardiac malignancy/infiltrative disease (e.g. cardiac amyloid).

The diagnosis may be suspected on the basis of pulse palpation, and is confirmed by electrocardiography.

Classification
AF should be classified according to the following categories:
- first presentation or recurrent
- self-terminating or non-self-terminating
- paroxysmal (self-terminating within 7 days)
- persistent (if it is cardioverted to sinus rhythm by any means, or lasts for more than 7 days)
- permanent (if it does not terminate, or it recurs within 24 hours of termination)
- lone (absence of associated structural heart disease).

In addition to an ECG, patients should undergo additional supporting investigations as discussed below.

Clinical presentation
Both AF and atrial flutter are commonly an incidental finding in a completely asymptomatic patient. Other important presentations include the following:
- palpitations
- shortness of breath
- chest pain
- dizziness
- ankle swelling
- intercurrent infections
- stroke/transient ischaemic attack.

Patients who present with new (< 48 hours) atrial fibrillation with any of the following features must have prompt electrical (DC) cardioversion as a matter of urgency:

- chest pain (but if there is an acute MI, treat this first!)
- signs of heart failure
- systolic blood pressure < 90 mmHg
- impaired consciousness level.

Initial investigations

- **U&E.** Ensure that there is no electrolyte imbalance responsible (Na^+ and K^+ levels are particularly important). Check urea and creatinine levels, as renal failure can cause AF. If the patient is uraemic, they may require dialysis (especially if they have uraemic pericarditis).
- **Bone profile.** Calcium should be checked and replaced or reduced as necessary.
- **Magnesium.** Electrolyte disturbances are a common cause of AF and are potentially reversible. Aim to keep magnesium levels above 1 mmol/l.
- **LFT.** This becomes particularly important if considering the initiation of amiodarone, which can result in a drug-induced hepatitis acutely, and in the chronic setting may cause cirrhosis.
- **Thyroid function.** Hypo- or hyperthyroidism is a potentially reversible cause of AF. Amiodarone may also result in thyroid dysfunction.
- **Chest X-ray.** Look for cardiomegaly, infection and pulmonary oedema.
- **Transthoracic echocardiography.** In addition to screening for underlying cardiac disease, this will include a measurement of left atrial size. If the latter is > 4 cm, this may confer additional thromboembolic risk, and also reduces the likelihood of restoring or maintaining sinus rhythm.
- **Septic screen.** If patients may have underlying infections or sepsis, a comprehensive screen should be sent. This should include a urine dip, urine MC&S, blood cultures, chest X-ray and, if applicable, stool cultures and wound swabs.
- Other investigations may be indicated, depending on the likely cause.

Further investigations
Holter monitors and Reveal® device
Patients with paroxysmal AF (PAF) may only be detected with longer-term

monitoring. Holter monitors are relatively commonplace, usually as a 24-hour tape. They can be used for a substantially longer period (e.g. 7 days). A Reveal® device can also be useful in some patients. Both of these methods of detecting arrhythmia may also be useful for assessing rate profiles and pauses.

Exercise ECG

This can be a useful test to determine whether rate control medication is adequate. Exercise-induced arrhythmias should be investigated in some circumstances. This is usually more applicable to ventricular arrhythmias.

Management

Emergency management of AF

Patients who demonstrate haemodynamic instability require DCCV under GA or conscious sedation. Do not attempt to do this without senior support. Ensure that the patient is kept nil by mouth. You will need to contact the following people urgently:

- anaesthetist
- cardiology registrar on call (or medical registrar if no cardiologists are available).

The patient must be on a cardiac monitor with regular blood pressure checks. If AF has been present for more than 48 hours, or the duration is unclear, any attempt at cardioversion must be preceded by TOE to exclude left atrial appendage thrombus which could be dislodged by a cardioversion and cause a stroke.

Non-emergency management of AF

Treatment for chronic AF has changed considerably over the last 10 years, and it is now recognised that there is no survival benefit for patients in sinus rhythm so long as they have had their thromboembolic risk calculated and addressed. This is achieved using the CHADS2 scoring system:

- Cardiac failure   score   1
- Hypertension   score   1
- Age > 75 years   score   1
- Diabetes mellitus   score   1
- Stroke or TIA   score   2

A total score of 0 indicates low risk. Aspirin 75 mg alone confers sufficient thromboembolic protection. Some physicians advocate higher doses of aspirin.

A total score of 1 indicates moderate risk. Aspirin or warfarin should be given, and the risks and benefits of each drug must be discussed with the patient.

A score of 2–6 indicates high risk. Warfarin thromboprophylaxis is recommended unless there are strong grounds for not using this treatment.

When considering warfarin, it is important to consider bleeding and the risk of falls, and to counsel the patient appropriately. The majority of patients can be started on warfarin in the outpatient setting; liaise with your local anticoagulation clinic. Some subsets of very high-risk patients, such as those with new (non-cerebral) embolus, or severe valvular or structural heart disease, may require inpatient anticoagulation.

In the context of acute stroke/TIA and AF, most neurologists recommend waiting for a period of at least 2 weeks before commencing full anticoagulation, in order to avoid the risk of haemorrhagic transformation. Aspirin is usually stopped once the warfarin dose is adequate (i.e. when the INR is 2–3). In the case of patients who have a strong indication for aspirin and clopidogrel (e.g. recent stent), ask for senior advice.

Rate control or rhythm control
A decision then needs to be made about whether to implement a rate or rhythm control strategy, and this mainly depends upon the symptoms. If the patient is very symptomatic with the following, it may be preferable to control the rhythm:
- palpitations
- breathlessness
- chest pain
- fatigue.

Up to 30% of patients with AF are asymptomatic, and it may therefore be appropriate to consider rhythm control. This can be broadly divided into the following types:
- pharmacological
- electrical
- invasive electrophysiological.

Pharmacological intervention
Several drugs can be used to treat AF. This book only deals with those most likely to be encountered by a foundation doctor. It must be remembered that all anti-arrhythmic drugs may also be pro-arrhythmic, and combinations of drugs may have unpredictable effects.

Rhythm control

Drugs that are used to restore sinus rhythm include the following.

- **Amiodarone.** This can be an effective drug, but it has several potentially severe side-effects, including photosensitivity reactions, corneal microdeposits, hepatic and thyroid toxicity, and pulmonary fibrosis. These tend to be cumulative and problematic with long-term use. Amiodarone can also cause severe reactions if extravasated, so should be administered with extreme caution if given peripherally. Amiodarone has a very long half-life (> 1 month), so even when it has been discontinued the effects will persist for some time.

- **Dronedarone.** This new drug is structurally related to amiodarone, but has a much smaller volume of distribution and a shorter elimination half-life (13–19 hours), has NYHA class I, II, III and IV actions, is a safer alternative than amiodarone for atrial fibrillation/atrial flutter, and is contraindicated in severe or recently decompensated symptomatic heart failure. It is currently being appraised by NICE for use in the UK. Dronedarone should be used as a second-line agent, after beta-blockers.

- **Flecainide.** This is a class Ic agent that affects sodium channels. It can be used both intravenously and orally, in acute and chronic AF. However, it should only be used in people with structurally normal hearts, as it can cause life-threatening ventricular arrhythmias. In practice, any patient with a history of any cardiac condition should not receive flecainide without expert advice.

- **Sotalol.** This has both class II and III effects. It is used less frequently in current practice.

Rate control

A resting heart rate target of < 90 beats/min should be set.

- **Beta-blockers.** These act on β1-receptors in the heart, and slow both the sinus node rate and conduction in the atrio-ventricular node. Metoprolol is a short-acting beta-blocker which is useful in beta-blocker-naive patients to check for potential side-effects. It can be switched to a longer-acting preparation once tolerance is known. If the patient has heart failure, prescribe a beta-blocker that is licensed for use in CCF (metoprolol, carvedilol and bisoprolol are common choices).

- **Calcium-channel blockers.** A variety of different preparations exist with varying duration of action. Familiarise yourself with this area

before prescribing. Calcium-channel blockers have varying degrees of negative inotropy, and should be used with caution in CCF patients.
  — **Verapamil.** This acts by slowing AV nodal conduction. It should not be co-administered with beta-blockers except under cardiology advice, due to the risk of excessive AV nodal block.
  — **Diltiazem.** This also slows AV conduction, but often to a lesser degree than verapamil.
- **Digoxin.** This is a cardiac glycoside with a weak positive inotropic effect. It slows AV conduction, but has a poor rate response so is not useful for active patients. Its use should be restricted to elderly or relatively immobile patients.

Some patients with AF are relatively bradycardic without the use of negatively chronotropic drugs. Holter monitoring is advisable, and permanent single chamber pacing may be indicated.

Electrical intervention
A synchronised DC shock can restore sinus rhythm in a significant number of patients. Factors that increase the likelihood of success include the following:
- shorter duration of AF
- absence of structural heart disease
- potentially reversible cause (e.g. sepsis).

It is important that the following steps are followed:
- documented INR > 2 for at least 4 weeks prior to DCCV
- potassium level > 3.5 mmol/l
- nil by mouth for > 6 hours.

If any of the following are present, discuss the case with the cardiology specialist registrar or consultant before proceeding:
- known intracardiac thrombus
- significant electrolyte imbalance
- digoxin toxicity
- cardiogenic shock
- refractory pulmonary oedema
- uncontrolled thyrotoxicosis
- permanent pacemaker
- pregnancy

- any condition that renders the patient incapable of giving informed consent
- any other condition that is thought to increase the risk of the procedure.

Informed consent must be obtained with the following specifics:
- risk of stroke < 1%
- risk of anaesthesia
- procedural failure
- skin erythema/burns.

The procedure can be summarised as follows.
1 Place pads in the AP position with a hands-free defibrillator, or in the right infraclavicular and apical position if using a paddle defibrillator (AP positioning is a useful pad position to try if the infraclavicular and apical position is unsuccessful).
2 Ensure that the shock is synchronised to the R-wave of the surface ECG.
3 Anaesthesia must be administered by an appropriately trained healthcare professional.
4 Record rhythm strip.
5 Deliver the minimum number of shocks required to achieve sinus rhythm as follows. Some centres advocate lower energies initially. However, others suggest delivering shocks at 200 J from the start (consult local guidelines). Consider using higher monophasic energy levels (360 J) if BMI is > 25 kg/m^2.
6 Record the duration of any sinus pauses, ventricular premature complexes, ST-segment deviation, recurrence of AF and significant atrioventricular block.
7 Record a heart rhythm strip after the procedure.
8 Document any complications.

If the patient has not been anticoagulated or has a subtherapeutic INR, TOE can be performed beforehand to exclude thrombus in the left atrial appendage prior to DC cardioversion.

Electrophysiological intervention
Atrial fibrillation
Catheter ablation of atrial fibrillation continues to improve. This is only performed in specialist centres by cardiac electrophysiologists, and it involves electrically isolating the pulmonary veins in the left atrium where the majority of AF originates. It is only indicated for very symptomatic patients, and

often a trial of alternative therapy is offered first to determine whether the patient feels better in sinus rhythm.

A permanent pacemaker and subsequent catheter AV nodal ablation is a palliative procedure that is used in extreme cases, as it renders the patient pacemaker-dependent.

Atrial flutter

This atrial arrhythmia arises due to a macro-re-entrant circuit within the right atrium (in 90% of cases), although several forms exist. It is usually associated with structural heart disease. Radio-frequency catheter ablation is curative, and should now be the first-line treatment in suitable patients. Referral to the cardiology team is therefore indicated. Drug treatment for flutter is often suboptimal, using the same drugs as described above. Anticoagulation is the same as for AF.

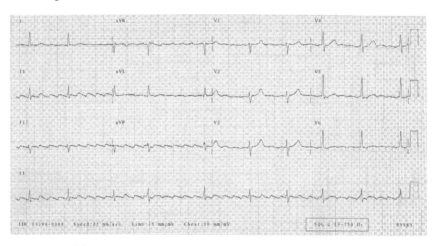

FIGURE 9.1 ECG showing atrial flutter with variable block.

Focal atrial tachycardia

This is due to a group of atrial cells firing more rapidly than the SA node, depolarising the myocardium and instigating a clinical tachycardia. They are classically paroxysmal with fast atrial rates. RFA should be offered in suitable patients. Rate-slowing calcium-channel blockers or beta-blockers can be used to control the ventricular rate.

Important tips

Previous echocardiograms

Look back to see whether the patient has had an echocardiogram. If they have a significantly enlarged left atrium, it is highly unlikely that it will be possible to restore sinus rhythm. These patients will be more effectively treated by rate control.

Old notes

Patients may have had previous different treatment trials, which may influence what treatment options are available for each individual patient. It is also important to look back and see whether they have undergone previous DCCV or ablation procedures.

Anticoagulation

Once the decision has been made that a patient requires anticoagulation with warfarin, it is the hospital team's responsibility to ensure that this has been properly explained to the patient and that they have appropriate follow-up to monitor their INR. If the patient is to be discharged before they have a therapeutic INR, ensure that they are on low-molecular-weight heparin until the INR comes into range. This may mean teaching the patient to self-administer the injections, or organising a district nurse. The patient must be advised to carry a card stating that they are on warfarin, and should inform other healthcare professionals, such as dentists. They should also know that other drugs, such as antibiotics, may interfere with their warfarin dosing.

Information to have to hand for ward rounds

1 An ECG demonstrating the patient's arrhythmia.
2 A post-procedure ECG to demonstrate sinus rhythm (if post RFA/DCCV/chemical cardioversion).
3 A 24-hour tape, or any other Holter monitor results.
4 Echocardiogram report.
5 Up-to-date bloods, including electrolytes and INR. The past 4 weeks of INR values are needed if the patient is to have elective DCCV.
6 Current and previous pharmacological regimens.
7 Observation chart for haemodynamic status.

Further reading

Relevant NICE guidelines (http://guidance.nice.org.uk):
- *Atrial Fibrillation*. CG 36. June 2006.

10

Tachyarrhythmias

Cardiac electrophysiology is an extensive area in cardiology, a detailed discussion of which is beyond the scope of this book. Here we shall consider some of the more important and common tachyarrhythmias that a junior doctor may encounter.

Aetiology

Fast heart rhythms can originate from the ventricles or atria (supraventricular). They usually indicate an underlying electrical or mechanical problem with cardiac conduction. At a tissue level there may be ischaemia, fibrosis (scarring) and infiltration of the heart muscle. Arrhythmias can also arise in a structurally normal heart, where genetics becomes important in the aetiology.

Tachyarrhythmias are classified according to their site of origin, whether above or below the AV node.

Ventricular arrhythmias: broad complex

Ventricular fibrillation

This is disorganised electrical activity with a fast rate, usually more than 300 beats/min.

Ventricular tachycardia

- Non-sustained VT consists of three or more beats, lasting less than 30 seconds.
- Sustained VT lasts for more than 30 seconds.

It is important to decide whether it is monomorphic (i.e. with the same QRS morphology) or polymorphic (i.e. with changing QRS morphology).

The axis and morphology will indicate the source of the tachycardia:

- LBBB pattern – arising from right ventricle
- RBBB pattern – arising from left ventricle.

Torsades de pointe

This is a particular type of VT associated with a classical twisting pattern on the ECG or rhythm strip (see Figure 10.1). It is associated with a prolonged QT interval. Potassium and magnesium replacement is required to reduce the QT interval. Ventricular pacing may be required while the metabolic status is abnormal.

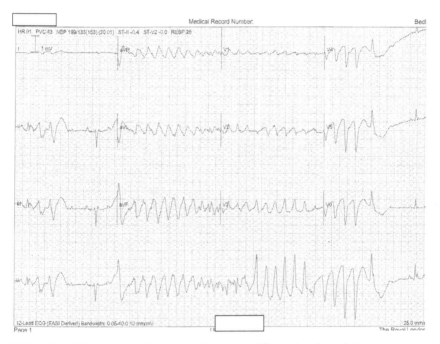

FIGURE 10.1 ECG showing the alternating axis of Torsades de pointe.

Supraventricular tachycardia (SVT): narrow complex

Atrio-ventricular nodal re-entry tachycardia (AVNRT)

AVNRT originates from above the ventricles. Instead of the electrical signal passing from the atria to the ventricle via the bundle of His, a re-entry circuit forms near the AV node (see Figure 10.2). AVNRT is the commonest SVT, and is most prevalent in women aged 20–30 years. It is usually characterised by an abrupt onset and offset. It may be triggered by stress, caffeine or alcohol.

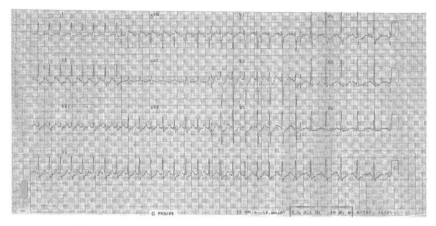

FIGURE 10.2 ECG showing AVNRT.

Atrio-ventricular re-entry tachycardia (AVRT)

AVRT originates from above the ventricles, like AVNRT. The electrical signal is transmitted from the atria to the ventricle via an accessory pathway, rather than via the AV node (hence the name AVRT). Wolff–Parkinson–White syndrome is a typical example, and the specific accessory pathway is called the bundle of Kent.

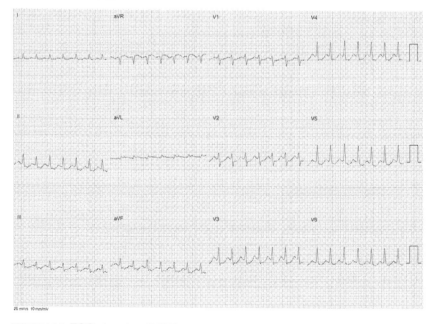

FIGURE 10.3 ECG showing AVRT.

Atrial fibrillation and atrial flutter

These are other common forms of supraventricular tachyarrhythmia, which are covered in detail in Chapter 9.

Diagnosis

Establish whether the tachyarrhythmia is haemodynamically stable or unstable.

- What is the patient's level of consciousness?
- What is their blood pressure?

If the patient is not conscious, follow the current UK resuscitation guidelines, and assess the patient using the ABC method. Put out a cardiac arrest call if necessary.

If possible try to obtain a 12-lead ECG, or at least ensure that the cardiac monitor can print a record of the rhythm. This will be useful later for confirming the diagnosis and guiding further management. In addition, consider the underlying diagnosis, as this may also require urgent treatment:

- myocardial infarction or coronary disease
- pulmonary embolus
- heart failure
- congenital heart disease
- cardiomyopathy
- ion-channel disease (long QT syndrome, Brugada syndrome, etc.)
- electrolyte disturbance, endocrine disturbance, drugs or toxins.

Initial investigations

These are often delayed until after treatment has been given, especially in the case of VT or VF. A routine work-up should cover the same investigations as discussed in Chapter 9, with the addition of the following:

- **Cardiac enzymes.** Myocardial infarction can result in arrhythmia. Infarcts involving the right coronary artery are more commonly associated with arrhythmia.
- **ECG.** A 12-lead ECG of the arrhythmia should be obtained, in addition to subsequent ECGs once the arrhythmia has been treated. ECGs can change quickly, so it is important to record them at regular intervals. Repolarisation changes may resolve with time. If possible, leave the ECG stickers on the patient's chest so lead positioning is consistent.
- **Echocardiogram.** Look for evidence of structural heart disease.

- **Holter monitoring and telemetry.** This usually involves 24-hour recording, but may be up to 7 days. It provides data from a 3-lead ECG, and is useful for investigating paroxysmal arrhythmias or the frequency of ectopics.

Further investigations

It is not always necessary to investigate all tachyarrhythmias further. The initial investigations may be adequate for obtaining the diagnosis.

Urinary catecholamines

Phaeochromocytoma can cause tachycardias with dramatic variations in blood pressure. Catecholamines are usually collected for 24 hours over 3 days. Discuss this with the laboratory so that they can provide the correct collection containers.

Exercise testing

Identify exercise-induced arrhythmias or ECG changes that suggest myocardial ischaemia.

Coronary angiography

This is used to evaluate new or old coronary artery disease.

Cardiac MRI

Arrhythmias arising in a structurally normal heart require further imaging. An MRI can detect scarring in the heart as well as conditions such as myocarditis, sarcoid, amyloid or previous infarction.

Electrophysiological study

This is an invasive test in which catheters are placed inside the heart. An electrical map is created to identify areas of abnormal conduction (*see* Figure 10.4). Drugs may be given to precipitate arrhythmias.

Reveal® device

This is a small device (about the size of a memory stick) that is implanted under the skin and which can be activated by the patient to store cardiac rhythms.

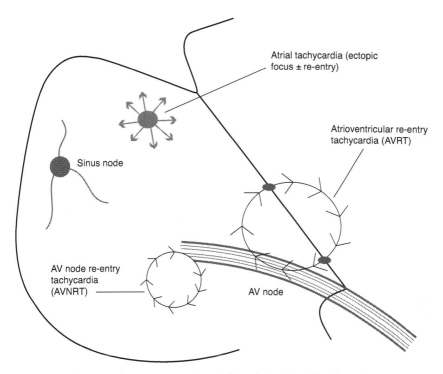

FIGURE 10.4 Schematic representation of the origin of atrial tachyarrhythmias.

Management

Try to correct any underlying cause (e.g. metabolic or electrolyte derangement).

> *Warning: Wide QRS tachycardia should be assumed to be VT if the diagnosis is unclear. If there is haemodynamic compromise, treatment always consists of urgent electrical cardioversion.*

Drugs

Drugs can be used in the acute and chronic management of tachyarrhythmia. A detailed knowledge of the source of the arrhythmia is important when deciding on treatment. AV nodal blocking manoeuvres (valsalva, carotid sinus massage) and drugs (*see* Table 10.1) are only useful for terminating arrhythmias that involve the AV node (i.e. AVNRT and AVRT, but not AF and atrial flutter).

Always have a defibrillator on standby in case the patient's condition changes rapidly or external pacing is required.

TABLE 10.1 Pharmacological management of supraventricular and ventricular arrhythmia

	SUPRAVENTRICULAR	VENTRICULAR
First line	Adenosine is used to block AV conduction. It confirms that the arrhythmia is arising from the atria, and is useful for terminating AVNRT and AVRT. Give intravenously in incremental doses of 3 mg, 6 mg, 12 mg, etc. Avoid using it in patients with heart block, and use with caution in those with asthma	Amiodarone given intravenously may be effective in terminating monomorphic and polymorphic VT. Avoid using it if there is a known history of long QT syndrome
Other	Alternatives are beta-blockers or verapamil, which also slow AV conduction Flecainide and amiodarone may also be used	Lidocaine IV can be used, especially if there is underlying myocardial ischaemia or infarction. In polymorphic VT, beta-blockers may also be used *Note*: Rapid pacing can terminate VT (via temporary wire or the patient's ICD or pacemaker). If ischaemia is driving the VT, consider urgent angiography for revascularisation
Chronic	A single episode does not usually warrant treatment. In recurrent cases beta-blockers or verapamil may be used for prevention	Amiodarone, sotolol or beta-blockers are useful for reducing VT in patients with LV dysfunction or poorly tolerated VT. Prophylactic anti-arrhythmic drugs are not useful in asymptomatic NSVT

Electrical cardioversion

This may be used to treat any tachyarrhythmia (except sinus tachycardia). In an unconscious or haemodynamically compromised patient this is the first-line treatment. If the patient is tolerating the tachyarrhythmia they will need sedation and/or anaesthesia first.

Ablation

Radio-frequency ablation is a permanent method of treating tachyarrhythmia. A catheter is placed inside the heart and radio-frequency energy is used to destroy the abnormal electrical pathways. The procedure is performed for all types of arrhythmias, but is most successful and low risk for AVNRT and AVRT. Cryoablation (freezing the tissue) is another method used to treat SVTs that originate from near the AV node.

Ventricular tachyarrhythmia may also be treated by ablation, but this is higher risk and less successful. Patients with monomorphic VT that is not treated with drugs gain most benefit.

Defibrillators

ICDs may be implanted in patients who have survived a cardiac arrest or who are considered at high risk of future ventricular arrhythmias. There are strict NICE guidelines on who is eligible:

- survivor of VF/VT cardiac arrest
- symptomatic VT (syncope or severe haemodynamic compromise)
- ejection fraction < 35% and NSVT
- ejection fraction < 30% and QRS duration > 120 ms
- high-risk familial or congenital heart disease.

Prognosis

SVTs are generally considered to be benign, but symptoms can have quite an intrusive effect on everyday life. Ablation is successful in up to 90% of patients with AVNRT, thus offering a curative treatment. Implantable defibrillators have improved the prognosis for patients with ventricular arrhythmias. However, there are other problems associated with their use, such as device failure, infection and inappropriate shocks.

Further reading

- DVLA Guidelines. *At a Glance Guide to the Current Medical Standards of Fitness to Drive.* DVLA; 2011. www.dft.gov.uk/dvla/medical/ataglance.aspx
- NICE Guidelines. *Implantable cardioverter defibrillators (ICDs) for the treatment of arrhythmias.* NICE; January 2006, reviewed July 2007. http://guidance.nice.org.uk/TA95/Guidance/pdf/English
- American College of Cardiology, American Heart Association and European Society of Cardiology. *Ventricular Arrhythmias and the Prevention of Sudden Cardiac Death.* ACC, AHA and ESC; 2006.

11

Bradyarrhythmias

Heart block

First-degree heart block

ECG diagnosis is made by demonstrating prolongation of the PR interval to > 200 ms. It very rarely requires specific intervention and has an excellent prognosis.

Causes
- May be a normal finding in young people.
- AV nodal disease.
- Vagal tone.
- Acute inferior MI.
- Myocarditis.
- Electrolyte disturbance.
- Drugs.

Second-degree heart block

There are two types of second-degree heart block, which differ greatly with regard to their management.

Mobitz I (also known as Wenckebach)
- Progressive PR lengthening, followed by 'dropped' beat.
- Usually disease of AV node.
- Rarely degenerates to malignant rhythms.
- May be found in asymptomatic young people.

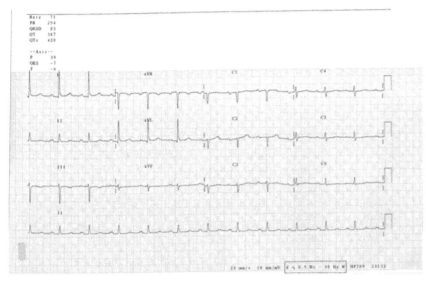

FIGURE 11.1 First-degree heart block. Note also P mitrale which is indicative of raised left atrial pressures.

Mobitz II

- Dropped beats, fixed ratio of P to QRS (2:1, 3:1, etc.).
- Usually disease of His or Purkinje fibres.
- May result in cardiac pauses, third-degree block, Stokes–Adams attacks or cardiac arrest.

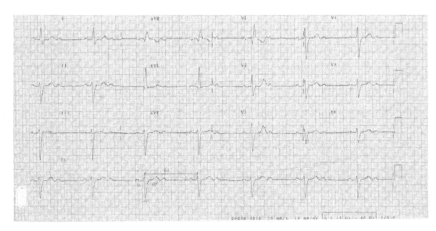

FIGURE 11.2 ECG showing Mobitz II 2:1 heart block.

Bifascicular block

- This is defined as the combination of RBBB, left axis deviation or LBBB and right axis deviation. If there is also first-degree heart block in the context of bifascicular block, it is termed trifascicular block.
- May be associated with a higher degree of block (a 24-hour tape is useful here).
- If associated with symptoms of dizziness/pre-syncope or syncope, a PPM should be offered.

Third-degree 'complete' heart block

- No fixed relationship of P to QRS.
- The 'escape rhythm' can be nodal or ventricular with its own native depolarisation rate (often slow rates).
- Exercise intolerance and ischaemic symptoms.

Causes

- MI affecting septum (inferior/anterior).
- Drugs (anti-arrhythmics, digoxin).
- Metabolic disturbance (hyperkalaemia).
- Cardiomyopathy (Lyme disease, acute rheumatic fever).

Junctional rhythm

- This refers to heart rhythms that originate from the 'junction' of the atria and ventricles.

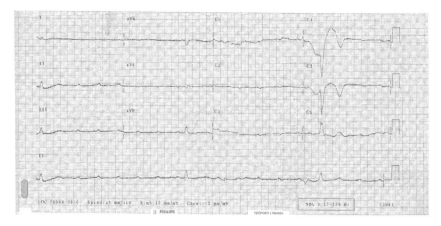

FIGURE 11.3 ECG showing complete AV dissociation is complete heart block.

- As such, no definite P-waves are present, but the rhythm tends to be regular.
- May be associated with tachycardia.
- May cause escape rhythm during bradycardia.

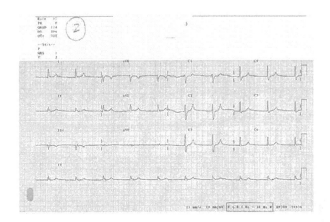

FIGURE 11.4 Junctional bradycardia, probably due to sinus node dysfunction. Note the absence of P-waves.

Sick sinus syndrome

This term refers to a spectrum of disorders encompassing sinus bradycardia, sinus arrest (pauses) and brady-tachy syndrome. The last diagnosis is made in the presence of both sinus bradycardia and pauses with evidence of atrial tachyarrhythmias.

Carotid sinus syndrome

Pressure on the carotid artery at the point at which it bifurcates can produce bradycardia and hypotension. This is the rationale behind carotid sinus massage. If a pause of > 3 seconds is provoked *and symptoms are reproduced*, this is an indication for pacing. This should only be performed under supervision, with appropriate electrocardiographic monitoring. The carotid arteries should be auscultated first to exclude a bruit, as pressure in the context of atherosclerotic disease may precipitate a stroke.

Vasovagal syncope

This diagnosis is usually obvious from the history, and there are very few indications for a pacemaker, which must be discussed with a cardiologist.

Initial investigations

A thorough understanding of the 12-lead ECG is of paramount importance in the diagnosis and management of arrhythmia. If you are unsure, always ask a senior, or even send a fax to a cardiologist for an opinion. A routine work-up should cover the same investigations as discussed in Chapter 9, with the addition of the following:

• **Ambulatory Holter monitoring.** This is designed to capture arrhythmia over time periods ranging from 24 hours to 1 week.

Management

If a bradyarrhythmia is associated with haemodynamic compromise, treat according to ALS guidelines.

A useful drug that is not included in the ALS algorithm is salbutamol. Although it is normally used in the treatment of asthma, the beta-agonist effect can on occasion be useful when treating bradycardic patients. In cases of difficult intravenous access this drug can be nebulised. It can also lower potassium so avoid if hypokalaemia is present.

If a bradyarrhythmia is well tolerated, there is more time in which to formulate a management plan. Always try to obtain documentary evidence of the arrhythmia, even if it is just a printout from a cardiac monitor on the ward, as this is invaluable to the cardiologist.

Drug history

Check for any rate-slowing medication that the patient may be taking, including less obvious drugs such as eye-drops for glaucoma that contain beta-blockers. These medications will often require either dose reduction or discontinuation.

Electrolytes

Correct any biochemical abnormalities, especially potassium and magnesium levels.

Temporary pacing

Temporary pacing can be achieved either transcutaneously or by inserting a pacing wire through a transvenous sheath in a large vein (usually the femoral, jugular or subclavian vein). Transvenous pacing used to be carried out by general medical registrars, but current guidelines recommend insertion only by cardiologists or other appropriately trained specialists, due to the high rate of complications.

Permanent pacing

Many bradyarrhythmias are treatable by insertion of a permanent pacemaker. This procedure is performed under conscious sedation by cardiologists. Implant technique is beyond the scope of this book, but essentially involves the positioning of one or two wires transvenously in the right atrium and/ or ventricle, and connection to a generator placed in a pocket fashioned in a pre-pectoral plane.

Permanent pacemaker implantation is indicated in Mobitz type II second-degree heart block, and in third-degree heart block, as well as in certain circumstances in patients with sick sinus syndrome, carotid sinus syndrome, vasovagal syncope, GUCH, and hypertrophic cardiomyopathy with LVOT obstruction. Referral to your local cardiologist is recommended.

Further reading

- www.escardio.org/guidelines-surveys/esc-guidelines/Pages/cardiac-pacing-and-cardiac-resynchronisation-therapy.aspx
- Epstein AE, DiMarco JP, Blenbogen KA *et al.* ACC/AHA/HRS 2008 guidelines for device-based therapy of cardiac rhythm abnormalities. *J Am Coll Cardiol.* 2008; **51:** 1–62.

It is also worth familiarising yourself with the rules about driving in relation to arrhythmias. These can be found at www.dvla.gov.uk/media/pdf/medical/aagv1.pdf

12

Valvular heart disease

Valvular heart disease is common. Diagnosis and management should be based on evaluation of symptoms, clinical examination and investigations. Patients are often asymptomatic or have modified their lifestyle to cope with slowly progressive symptoms. It is essential to consider endocarditis if there has been a rapid clinical change. A change in murmur should be investigated.

Epidemiology

Aortic stenosis is the most common form of valvular heart disease, and tends to present in patients aged between 60 and 80 years, although it can present at any age. Around 2–7% of the population aged over 65 years have some degree of aortic stenosis, with a male preponderance.

The most common mitral valve lesion is mitral regurgitation. Mitral valve prolapse occurs in around 5% of the normal population, but is associated with other conditions such as HOCM, Ehlers–Danlos syndrome and Marfan syndrome. Although the exact incidence of mitral stenosis is unknown, it is much less common than mitral regurgitation and mitral valve prolapse. The incidence has fallen significantly in the western world as a result of the decreasing incidence of rheumatic fever.

Right-sided valvular heart disease can be congenital, secondary to left heart disease or endocarditis, or a result of lung pathology causing cor pulmonale.

Aortic stenosis

Aetiology

Age of presentation plays a significant role in the likely aetiology. In the elderly it is predominantly calcific or degenerative, whereas in the young it is more likely to be congenital due to a bicuspid valve. Although it is increasingly uncommon in the western world, rheumatic valvular disease still occurs.

Clinical presentation
Presentation can vary enormously, and in some instances patients are completely asymptomatic, the diagnosis being made by the incidental finding of a murmur.

History
The following important areas within the history have prognostic significance:
- angina – 50% mortality at 5 years
- syncope – 50% mortality at 3 years
- breathlessness – 50% mortality at 2 years.

Exercise tolerance will often have decreased. However, the patient may be unaware of this at first as they adapt their life within these limitations. Important points to cover when enquiring about exercise tolerance should include the following:
- How far can the patient walk on the flat and on an incline?
- Can they manage to walk up stairs?
- What could they do 6 months or a year ago?
- Have they had to stop any activities that they used to enjoy?
- What limits their exercise tolerance (breathlessness, pain, fatigue, other reasons)?

Enquire about childhood infection with rheumatic fever, and what symptoms they experienced. Also ask about rectal blood loss in anaemic patients, as there is an association between aortic stenosis and angiodysplasia (Heyde's syndrome).

Examination
Classically on examination there is an ejection systolic murmur which radiates to the carotid arteries. The loudness is *not* related to severity. In fact in severe AS the murmur is often quiet and S2 is inaudible due to restricted valve motion. It may be difficult to hear the murmur in the setting of heart failure. Clinical markers of severity include the following:
- narrow pulse pressure
- palpable thrill in the aortic area
- soft S2

- long murmur
- delayed A2 or reversed splitting of heart sounds.

Patients may later develop signs of right heart failure secondary to left heart failure.

Investigations
- **FBC.** Anaemia may contribute to symptoms such as angina and breathlessness, and should always be investigated further.
- **U&E.** Renovascular disease often coexists. Furthermore, patients are likely to require nephrotoxic drugs, and will inevitably require coronary angiography if valve replacement is to be considered.
- **Chest X-ray.** Calcification in the aorta may be observed. Look for signs of heart failure and cardiomegaly.
- **ECG.** Look for left ventricular hypertrophy with or without a strain pattern, left axis deviation and repolarisation changes (often T-wave inversion in the inferolateral leads).
- **Transthoracic echocardiogram.** This will usually clarify the diagnosis. Look for the following features:
  — gradient (mean gradient > 40 mmHg is severe)
  — aortic valve area (area < 1 cm^2 is severe)
  — LV function and LV size
  — LV wall thickness
  — LVEF – if LV function is poor it is easy to underestimate the severity of stenosis, as cardiac output is low and the velocity of blood flow through the aortic valve will be reduced. In this situation, exercise stress echo or an invasive assessment of the AV pressure gradient may be warranted.
- **Exercise testing.** This may also be helpful to objectively assess functional capacity in patients who appear to have asymptomatic severe aortic stenosis. This must be discussed with a cardiologist, as severe aortic stenosis is a contraindication to exercise testing unless supervised by experts.

Management
Medical management
Some patients may not initially require any active management, but will need serial clinical and echocardiographic follow-up. It may be that they later require referral for surgical intervention.

Optimisation of medical therapies such as ACEi, beta-blockers and diuretics is commonly initiated, although there is no consensus that these slow the progression of aortic stenosis. Vasodilators (including ACEi) and strenuous exertion should be avoided in severe aortic stenosis, as these will increase the trans-valvular gradient.

Surgical management

Surgery is indicated if any of the following are present:

- severe aortic stenosis and any symptoms
- severe aortic stenosis undergoing CABG, aortic or other valve surgery
- asymptomatic severe aortic stenosis and LVEF < 50%
- asymptomatic severe aortic stenosis and symptoms or fall in blood pressure on exercise
- moderate aortic stenosis and any symptoms.

Percutaneous aortic valve replacement is increasing in popularity, and outcomes in tertiary centres are comparable with those achieved by surgery. Current indications are those where surgery is high risk (EuroSCORE > 20%), contraindicated or technically challenging (e.g. thoracic deformity, previous CABG, porcelain aorta).

Prognosis

Predictors of progression include age, atherosclerosis, calcified valve and exercise intolerance. Poor LV function and symptoms of heart failure are associated with the worst prognosis.

Aortic regurgitation

Aetiology

There are multiple causes, the most common being an abnormal valve (e.g. bicuspid aortic valve) or abnormal aortic root (due to hypertension, Marfan syndrome, etc.). It is important to exclude endocarditis and type A aortic dissection in new cases of acute aortic regurgitation.

History

This is likely to vary significantly. In the acute setting, the main symptoms are as follows:

- aortic dissection:
  - sudden tearing inter-scapular pain
  - pain maximal at onset
  - may be accompanied by vagal or syncopal symptoms

  — possible neurological features with hemiparesis if dissection involves
    the origin of the carotid artery
- endocarditis:
  — fevers
  — drenching night sweats
  — weight loss.

In the more chronic setting, patients may be either completely asymptomatic
or complain of the following:
- breathlessness
- orthopnoea and PND
- decreasing exercise tolerance
- angina (since there is reduced coronary perfusion during diastole).

Examination

On clinical examination there will often be signs of low diastolic pressure,
collapsing and prominent arterial pulsations and a diastolic murmur. In
the setting of endocarditis, evidence of conduction disease on the ECG
should raise suspicion of an aortic root abscess. Examine the patient for all
peripheral pulses in the context of aortic dissection.

  Clinical markers of severity include the following:
- wide pulse pressure (> 100 mmHg)
- low diastolic blood pressure (< 40 mmHg)
- collapsing pulse
- short murmur (in the acute setting only).

The mechanism and severity of aortic regurgitation should be assessed by
echocardiography, but be aware that the findings depend on the loading
conditions.

Investigations

The choice of investigations is likely to depend very much on the suspected
underlying cause, which will be largely dictated by a good-quality history.
- **FBC.** Anaemia may be the result of aortic dissection, endocarditis
  or another underlying process. Check that the WCC is not elevated,
  especially in the context of suspected endocarditis.
- **U&E.** Diuretics are often required, so it is important to ascertain the
  baseline renal function. In the acute setting of aortic dissection, renal
  function may deteriorate if the dissection extends to involve the renal
  arteries.

- **LFT.** Hepatic congestion may result from progression to heart failure, and cause deranged liver function tests.
- **CRP and ESR.** It is important to check inflammatory markers if endocarditis is suspected.
- **Clotting screen.** This is only required in the acute setting if aortic dissection is suspected, so that any clotting abnormalities can be corrected.
- **Blood cultures.** These are required if endocarditis is suspected (*see* Chapter 13).
- **Chest X-ray.** Look for features of heart failure and cardiomegaly. Look at the diameter of the mediastinum in suspected cases of aortic dissection.
- **Transthoracic echocardiogram.** Look for the following:
  — *mechanism*: tricuspid or bicuspid valve, annular dilatation, aortic root size
  — *consequences*: LV enlargement and LV function
  — *severity*: markers of severe aortic regurgitation include a broad regurgitant jet that extends far back into the left ventricle, and diastolic flow reversal in the descending aorta.

Management
Asymptomatic mild and moderate aortic regurgitation requires surveillance with annual clinical examination and echocardiography. Aortic root disease is usually monitored with serial CT or MRI. High blood pressure should be treated with ACE inhibitors or calcium-channel blockers.

Indications for surgery
- Severe aortic regurgitation:
  — symptomatic patients (angina or NHYA class II to IV)
  — asymptomatic patients with LVEF < 50% or those undergoing CABG or other surgery
  — asymptomatic patients with LVEF > 50% if LV is severely dilated (> 70 mm in diastole or > 50 mm in systole).
- Mild or moderate aortic regurgitation if there is evidence of aortic root disease:
  — > 45 mm in patients with Marfan syndrome
  — > 50 mm in patients with bicuspid aortic valve
  — > 55 mm in all others.

Prognosis

Acute aortic regurgitation (due to dissection or endocarditis) has a poor prognosis and usually requires surgical intervention. Asymptomatic severe aortic regurgitation has a reasonable prognosis so long as surgery is timed correctly. The prognosis is poor in the chronic group if surgery is delayed until the patient is symptomatic.

Mitral regurgitation

Aetiology

Mitral regurgitation is the second most common valvular lesion after aortic stenosis. As the prevalence of rheumatic heart disease is decreasing, most causes can be categorised as *structural* or *functional*.

- *Structural* causes include leaflet prolapse, chordal rupture, papillary muscle dysfunction, endocarditis and connective tissue disorders.
- *Functional* causes include dilated mitral annulus (which is common with IHD) and cardiomyopathy.

Clinical presentation

As with previous valvular abnormalities, the clinical presentation is dependent upon the underlying cause.

History

Acutely ill patients may give a history suggestive of underlying endocarditis or acute breathlessness having suffered a recent myocardial infarction (resulting in papillary muscle rupture). In the acute setting, patients often do not tolerate mitral regurgitation well, as the left atrium has not had sufficient time to dilate and accommodate the sudden change in pressure.

In the case of mild mitral regurgitation, patients are often completely asymptomatic, with the incidental finding of a murmur on clinical examination. Those who are symptomatic often give a history of the following:

- dyspnoea
- fatigue
- palpitations – this may be the result of coexisting atrial fibrillation, which is very commonly associated with mitral valve disease.

Examination

Clinical examination usually detects moderate and severe mitral regurgitation. Patients may have a displaced and hyperdynamic apex beat, irregularly irregular pulse (AF), right ventricular heave, and a pansystolic murmur that radiates to the axilla.

Clinical markers of severity include the following:

- soft S1
- third heart sound (rapid ventricular filling from the left atrium, and excludes significant mitral stenosis)
- wide splitting of S2 (caused by early closure of the aortic valve as the LV empties earlier).

Investigations

- **FBC.** Anaemia may be the result of endocarditis or another underlying process. Check that the WCC is not elevated, especially in the context of suspected endocarditis.
- **U&E.** Diuretics are likely to be required, and therefore a baseline level of renal function is important.
- **LFT.** Hepatic congestion may result from progression to heart failure and cause deranged liver function tests.
- **CRP and ESR.** It is important to check inflammatory markers if endocarditis is suspected.
- **Blood cultures.** If endocarditis is suspected, three sets of blood cultures should be taken from three different sites, ideally at least 1 hour apart. If possible this should be done while the patient is off antibiotics. However, in an acutely unwell patient, blood cultures should not delay treatment with antibiotics.
- **Chest X-ray.** Look for features of heart failure and cardiomegaly.
- **ECG.** Look for atrial fibrillation, which is commonly associated with mitral valve disease (more often with mitral stenosis). Also look for evidence of previous myocardial infarction which may have resulted in papillary muscle rupture.
- **Transthoracic echocardiogram.** Key parameters to look for on echo relate to the severity and consequences of mitral regurgitation:
  — the proximal isovelocity surface area (PISA) and regurgitant volume are the best indicators of severity
  — left atrial size and pulmonary artery pressure indicate the consequences of mitral regurgitation
  — LV function may be hyperdynamic to compensate for the lack of forward flow
  — regional wall motion abnormalities may indicate previous infarction
  — leaflet prolapse, aberrant chordae and annular calcification.
- A TOE is often required to more accurately assess the mechanism

of mitral regurgitation and its suitability for repair. It also allows visualisation of the left atrial appendage where a thrombus may form.

Management

Patients with asymptomatic and mild to moderate mitral regurgitation must be followed up with regular clinical examination and echocardiography. There is limited evidence for medical treatment in mitral regurgitation. However, vasodilators (nifedipine) and ACE inhibitors have been shown to improve symptoms and prevent progressive LV dilatation. Diuretics are the mainstay of treatment, to relieve breathlessness. Atrial fibrillation should be managed in the conventional way with rate control together with appropriate anticoagulation (in accordance with the NICE guidelines). Cardioversion (electrical or chemical) in the context of mitral valve disease should be discussed with a cardiologist.

The decision to proceed with surgery depends on the symptoms of the patient and the likelihood of success. Consideration must be given to whether the valve is repairable or must be replaced. Sometimes this ultimately depends on the skills and expertise of the surgeon. Indications for surgical repair include the following:

- symptomatic mitral regurgitation with LVEF < 30% and end systolic diameter (ESD) < 55 mm
- asymptomatic mitral regurgitation with LV dysfunction, ESD > 45 mm and/or LVEF < 60%
- asymptomatic mitral regurgitation with good LV function and atrial fibrillation or pulmonary hypertension > 50 mmHg at rest.

There is limited evidence for operating on patients with severe LV dysfunction, unless repair is likely to be feasible and they have no other comorbidities.

Mitral clip

Percutaneous procedures to treat mitral regurgitation are now being performed in specialist centres. These involve trans-septal puncture to access the left ventricle. Placement of one or more clips to join the anterior and posterior mitral valve leaflets can then be carried out to reduce the regurgitant orifice. This works best in functional mitral regurgitation.

Prognosis

Acute mitral regurgitation is poorly tolerated and carries a poor prognosis. In asymptomatic patients, chronic mitral regurgitation generally has a good prognosis. The mild form of the condition is common and requires no specific surveillance.

Right-sided valvular heart disease

Right-sided valvular disease is usually congenital, or is the result of left heart disease or occurs in the context of cor pulmonale, and rarely occurs in isolation. A detailed discussion is beyond the scope of this book, but we shall very briefly cover tricuspid regurgitation.

Tricuspid regurgitation

Severe tricuspid regurgitation is usually functional (due to right ventricular dysfunction) rather than structural (due to a problem with the valve itself). The exception to this is right-sided endocarditis causing valvular destruction (e.g. in intravenous drug abusers). The right ventricle can fail because of pressure overload (i.e. pulmonary hypertension of any cause) or volume overload (e.g. ASD or intrinsic RV disease).

Clinically, tricuspid regurgitation is detected by raised JVP, often visible at the ear lobes, and other signs of right heart failure (e.g. hepatomegaly, peripheral oedema, ascites).

Indications for surgery include the following:

- severe tricuspid regurgitation in a patient having mitral or aortic valve surgery
- severe primary tricuspid regurgitation without RV dysfunction.

Surgery for valve disease: general points

Metal vs. tissue valves

The decision as to whether to implant a tissue valve or a metal valve is based on a number of factors. Metal valves require long-term anticoagulation, but last longer than tissue valves. Tissue valves will need to be replaced after approximately 10 years. Therefore age, risk of re-operation and contraindications to long-term anticoagulation are considered. Patient choice is also important. Women of childbearing age who require valve replacement may wish to have a tissue valve implanted initially to avoid the teratogenic effects of warfarin, and then have a metallic valve implanted later when the tissue valve needs to be replaced.

Endocarditis

All patients with valvular heart disease are at risk of endocarditis. Antibiotics are no longer routinely recommended to prevent endocarditis, but a regular dental check-up and good dental hygiene are essential.

The EuroSCORE

This is used to predict operative mortality. It takes into account patient age, renal function, comorbidity and type of surgery planned. An online calculator can be found at www.euroscore.org

Further reading

- The Task Force on the Management of Valvular Heart Disease of the European Society of Cardiology. Guidelines on the management of valvular heart disease. *Eur Heart J.* 2007; **28**: 230–68.

13

Endocarditis

Epidemiology

The incidence is 1.7–6.2 per 100 000 person-years.

The risk increases with age, male gender and predisposing factors (e.g. intravenous drug use and structurally abnormal heart).

The demographic make-up of your local hospital catchment area will influence the number and distribution of cases seen.

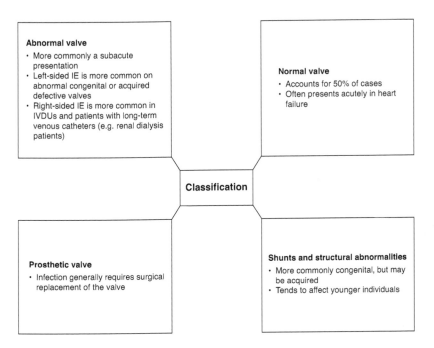

Abnormal valve
- More commonly a subacute presentation
- Left-sided IE is more common on abnormal congenital or acquired defective valves
- Right-sided IE is more common in IVDUs and patients with long-term venous catheters (e.g. renal dialysis patients)

Normal valve
- Accounts for 50% of cases
- Often presents acutely in heart failure

Classification

Prosthetic valve
- Infection generally requires surgical replacement of the valve

Shunts and structural abnormalities
- More commonly congenital, but may be acquired
- Tends to affect younger individuals

FIGURE 13.1

Right-sided infective endocarditis tends to be more common in IVDUs and patients with long-term venous catheters. As a result of venous seeding, the slower circulatory velocity contributes to risk by producing a longer contact time between infective organisms and cardiac tissue.

Aetiology

Relatively often, no organisms are cultured despite a diagnosis of infective endocarditis being made. Figure 13.2 shows the sites where these organisms are classically found.

Other organisms responsible include the following:
- HACEK organisms (*Haemophilus, Actinobacillus, Cardiobacterium, Eikenella* and *Kingella* species) are rare. If you want these to be tested for, you must specify this to the microbiologists, as it is not routine.
- Immunocompromised patients are susceptible to fungal causes of endocarditis (e.g. *Candida, Aspergillus*).

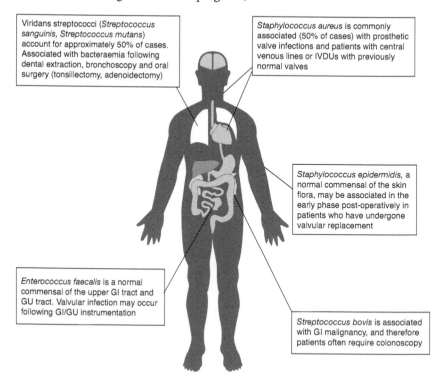

FIGURE 13.2 Causative organisms and their typical origin.

- Libman–Sacks endocarditis in SLE is a sterile endocarditis and is exceptionally rare.

Clinical presentation

It is important to document the presence or absence of the following features in your history and examination.

Systemic signs of infection

- Fevers.
- Malaise.
- Rigors.
- Night sweats.
- Weight loss.
- Anaemia.

Immune complex deposition

- Janeway lesions.
- Osler's nodes.
- Roth's spots (if retinal lesions are suspected, refer for a formal ophthalmological opinion).
- Splinter haemorrhages.
- Microscopic haematuria.

Valvular features

- New or changing murmur.
- Signs and symptoms of heart failure (*see* Box 13.1).
- Aortic valve IE:
  — prolonged PR interval may be seen as a result of aortic root abscess
  — PR prolongation occurs due to the proximity of the abscess to the conduction system of the heart.

Embolic phenomena

- Emboli may cause abscess formation in the brain/spinal cord, kidneys, liver, spleen, heart and GI tract with associated symptoms of each.
- Right-sided infective endocarditis may cause pulmonary abscess formation (look for cavities on chest X-ray).

> **BOX 13.1** Findings in left and right heart failure
>
> Left heart failure:
> - Shortness of breath on exertion
> - Orthopnoea (shortness of breath on lying flat)
> - Paroxysmal nocturnal dyspnoea (acute breathlessness that causes waking from sleep)
>
> Right heart failure:
> - Abdominal distension secondary to ascites
> - Pitting pedal oedema
> - Tenderness over the liver secondary to hepatic congestion

Initial investigations

- **FBC.** Normocytic anaemia, neutrophil leucocytosis, and thrombocytopenia in chronic disease.
- **CRP and ESR.** These are raised in inflammatory conditions as a non-specific finding.
- **U&E.** Renal function may be deranged secondary to immune complex deposition and/or increased insensible fluid loss due to pyrexia resulting in pre-renal failure.
- **LFT.** These may be abnormal, especially ALP and GGT, often secondary to hepatic congestion.
- **Immunology.** There is a polyclonal increase in serum immunoglobulins, reduced complement, and positive rheumatoid factor.
- **Urine dipstick.** If haematuria is present, send urine for MC&S and urinary casts. Haematuria occurs due to immune complex deposition resulting in glomerulonephritis. This inflammatory response causes destruction of the glomeruli, which are shed and appear as red cell casts in the urine. Consider a vasculitis screen (ANCA, ANA, rheumatoid factor, C3/C4 complement, anti-glomerular basement membrane (GBM) antibodies).
- **Clotting screen.** This is important, as the patient may need urgent surgery. They may also have deranged clotting secondary to sepsis or hepatic congestion which can result in malproduction of clotting factors.
- **ECG.** Look for signs of PR interval prolongation, which is itself a sign of aortic root abscess.

- **Chest X-ray.** Look for evidence of heart failure (*see* Figure 13.3 for typical features).
- **Fundoscopy.** Formal dilated fundoscopy to check for Roth's spots in the retinae.
- **TTE.** This should be booked as soon as endocarditis is suspected.

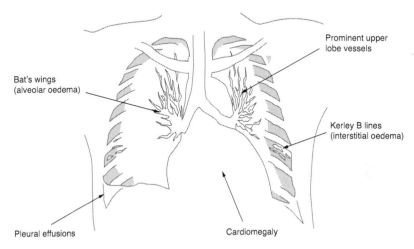

FIGURE 13.3 Typical features of heart failure on chest X-ray.

Further investigations

Blood cultures

Take three sets from three different sites over a 24-hour period. Each set must be taken at least 1 hour apart from the others. An aseptic technique is essential for this procedure. Ensure that the area from which the blood is taken is cleaned with a 70% alcohol swab, and that the tops of the bottles are also cleaned with alcohol swabs. Change the needle before filling the bottle with blood in order to minimise the risk of contamination. If you can make the diagnosis of endocarditis without blood cultures, *do not delay giving antibiotics*. Take all of the cultures together, as it is important to identify the causative organism.

Transthoracic echocardiogram

Look for abnormal valves, echogenic masses/vegetations on valves, new regurgitation and chamber size. With worsening aortic regurgitation the LV chamber dilates, and with worsening mitral regurgitation the LA chamber dilates.

Trans-oesophageal echocardiogram

TTE is often non-diagnostic for a variety of reasons, and TOE should then be considered if clinical suspicion remains high. This is an invasive procedure, and it must be discussed with a cardiology specialist registrar or consultant. TOE has a much higher sensitivity for visualising vegetations on the valves than TTE.

Complications of TOE include aspiration, haemorrhage, anaesthetic risk and oesophageal perforation. The cardiology registrar or consultant should obtain consent. Patients should be nil by mouth for 6 hours before the procedure. Because a local anaesthetic is used at the back of the throat, the patient must not consume hot food or drinks for 2 hours after the procedure, in order to prevent burns or aspiration.

Diagnostic criteria

The diagnosis of endocarditis is based on the Duke criteria, which are listed in Box 13.2.

BOX 13.2 Duke criteria for the diagnosis of endocarditis

Major criteria

1 Microbiological:
   - typical organisms in two separate cultures, *or*
   - persistently positive blood cultures (e.g. three positive cultures more than 12 hours apart).
2 Evidence of cardiac involvement:
   - positive echocardiogram (vegetations, abscess, new native or prosthetic valvular regurgitation).

Minor criteria

1 Predisposition to endocarditis (prosthetic valves, existing valvular disease, congenital heart disease, valvular prolapse, hypertrophic cardio-myopathy, IVDU).
2 Fever > 38 °C.
3 Vascular complications.
4 Immunological complications.
5 Positive blood cultures that do not meet the major criteria.

A definite diagnosis of endocarditis can be made with:
- two major Duke criteria, *or*
- one major Duke criterion plus three minor Duke criteria, *or*
- all five minor Duke criteria.

Management

Medical management

These patients should always be managed by cardiologists, together with prompt microbiological advice. It is important that three or more blood cultures are taken before initiation of antibiotic treatment, unless the patient becomes haemodynamically unstable. In these cases a cardiothoracic opinion is mandatory.

Initially, infective endocarditis is often managed with broad-spectrum antibiotics until a specific organism has been cultured and its antibiotic sensitivity is known. However, always consult your local hospital guidelines. When deciding which antibiotic to use, it is important to consider the patient's history and the likely causative organism. For example, it is likely that a different organism will be responsible in a patient who is an IVDU with suspected IE, compared with a patient who has recently undergone a bowel resection.

TABLE 13.1 Suggested initial empirical antibiotic therapy for infective endocarditis, which can be modified when the microbiological organisms are known (consult with local hospital guidelines)

PRESENTATION	ANTIBIOTIC REGIMEN
Gradual onset	Benzylpenicillin 2.4 g IV 4-hourly + gentamicin 3 mg/kg daily in one to three divided doses (check levels)
Acute onset	Flucloxacillin 2 g IV 6-hourly + gentamicin 3 mg/kg daily in one to three divided doses (check levels)
Recent prosthetic valve	Vancomycin 15 mg/kg IV 12-hourly infused over 60 minutes (check levels) + gentamicin 3 mg/kg daily in one to three divided doses (check levels) + rifampicin 300 mg by mouth 12-hourly (check LFT)
IVDU	Vancomycin 15 mg/kg IV 12-hourly infused over 60 minutes (check levels) + flucloxacillin 2 g IV 6-hourly

Surgical management

Surgical treatment should be considered in the following scenarios:
- Haemodynamic compromise secondary to valvular destruction.

- Failed medical management, as defined by no response or a suboptimal response to antibiotic therapy (persistent fever, changing or new murmur, etc.), relapsing infection, persistent fever, and worsening echo parameters of cardiac function.
- Consider early surgery for fungal and prosthetic valve endocarditis.
- Complications including intracardiac abscess, high-degree AV block, recurrent septic emboli, and perforation of intracardiac structures.

If a patient is to be considered for surgery, ensure that an appropriate pre-operative work-up has been arranged. This will consist of the following:
- dental check (unless the patient has false teeth)
- lung function testing.

Most centres routinely perform coronary angiography on these patients pre-operatively to determine whether there is coexisting coronary disease that requires treatment.

BOX 13.3 Daily monitoring and investigations

1 Close observations of vital signs.
2 Blood cultures whenever there is a temperature spike > 38 °C.
3 Daily examination looking specifically for any new peripheral stigmata of endocarditis or a changing and/or new murmur.
4 Daily urine dip. If the patient develops haematuria, they will need a full vasculitic screen.
5 Daily ECG to look for conduction abnormalities, particularly PR prolongation.
6 Daily bloods – FBC, U&E, CRP and ESR (LFT should be done twice a week if the patient is on rifampicin).
7 Therapeutic drug monitoring for antibiotic dosing as appropriate.

Important tips

Microbiology

Discuss the case with a microbiologist as soon as you suspect that a patient may have endocarditis. Early treatment with organism-specific antibiotics may be life-saving. Keep them updated about the patient's condition, as they may wish to change the antibiotics.

Cardiology

Discuss the case with cardiology early on, and ensure that you have carried out the initial investigations and booked the patient for a TTE. Cardiology will often take over the patient's care once a formal diagnosis has been made.

Cannulae

Intravenous cannulae are a common source of infection in hospitals. Ensure that you change the cannula every 3 days, and inspect cannula sites daily for early signs of local infection. Write the date of insertion on the cannula dressing, and record this in the notes to avoid confusion. If your patient is likely to require a prolonged course of antibiotics, you may wish to consider using a PICC line.

Previous records

Review the patient's case notes, looking in particular for details of previous echocardiograms as a comparison, and previously documented murmurs.

Future advice

Once a patient has been diagnosed with either an abnormal valve or endocarditis, it is important that they inform other healthcare professionals, such as their dentist. Once a valvular abnormality is present, there is a predisposition to infection of the valve. Infections may occur as a result of instrumentation, such as dental work, or future surgery.

Information to have to hand for ward rounds

1 Up-to-date bloods, including FBC, U&E, CRP and ESR.
2 Daily ECG, and a knowledge of what it shows.
3 Urine dipstick result.
4 Results of the most recent echocardiogram, or the date when echo is booked.
5 Up-to-date microbiology results.
6 Current antibiotic regimen and length of course to date.
7 Observation chart for temperature and haemodynamic status.

Further reading

- NICE Guidelines. *Antimicrobial prophylaxis against infective endocarditis.* NICE: March 2008. http://guidance.nice.org.uk/CG64

14

Hypertension

Epidemiology

Hypertension is extremely prevalent in the UK, and its incidence rises sharply with advancing age, such that around 50% of individuals aged over 65 years have this diagnosis.

Aetiology

Hypertension is very common, and is associated with a high cardiovascular and cerebrovascular risk. Both genetic and environmental factors contribute to the development of hypertension. Adults should be screened every 5 years, and those on treatment should have at least an annual check-up. The vast majority (approximately 90%) of hypertension is primary (essential) hypertension, with no identifiable cause.

Secondary causes of hypertension account for only around 10% of cases. However, they should still be considered in all new diagnoses, particularly in younger people.

Renovascular hypertension

Reduced renal blood flow can cause hypertension by activating the renin–angiotensin–aldosterone system, with subsequent salt and water retention. Increasing age and atherosclerosis are contributing factors. Renovascular hypertension should be suspected in patients with progressive renal failure, refractory hypertension (HTN), severe HTN, worsening of renal function with ACE inhibitors, recurrent pulmonary oedema or asymmetrical kidney size. Fibromuscular dysplasia is the commonest cause in young women.

Primary hyperaldosteronism (Conn's syndrome)

Aldosterone-producing tumours can cause secondary hypertension. Adenomas are more common than carcinomas, and are located in the adrenal glands. Conn's syndrome should be suspected in young or drug-refractory patients. A significant fall in potassium level with diuretics should raise the suspicion of underlying aldosterone excess. Patients may present with hypertension or symptoms of hypokalaemia (e.g. muscle cramps, polyuria, arrhythmias). Specialist function tests may be needed to confirm the diagnosis (e.g. renin and aldosterone levels, captopril or saline challenge). CT or MRI imaging of the adrenal glands should be performed.

Other secondary causes
- Drugs (NSAIDs, OCP, steroids, liquorice).
- Phaeochromocytoma (paroxysmal symptoms).
- Coarctation (radio-femoral delay or weak femoral pulses).
- Cushing's disease (general appearance).
- Carcinoid syndrome.
- Cerebrovascular causes (rare).

Clinical presentation

More commonly patients are completely asymptomatic, and are diagnosed with an incidental finding of hypertension. Patients may also present for the first time with the complications of hypertension. History and examination play an important role in the diagnosis of an underlying cause of hypertension.

Hypertensive crisis
- This is a term reserved for patients who present with usually acute hypertension resulting in end-organ damage. This is a medical emergency. It must be managed with senior advice, often on an HDU, ICU or CCU. Patients usually have a systolic blood pressure of > 200 mmHg and a diastolic blood pressure of > 120 mmHg.
- History is dependent on which end organs have been affected. Patients may present with headache, visual disturbance, confusion, chest pain, pulmonary oedema or renal failure.
- Examination may reveal focal neurology, papilloedema or pulmonary oedema.

Phaeochromocytoma

This is an adrenal neuroendocrine tumour that secretes catecholamines, thus causing hypertension. There are typically signs and symptoms of sympathetic nervous system activation (e.g. sweating, flushing, tachycardia). Up to 25% of cases are familial.

Aortic coarctation

This describes a focal aortic narrowing, which is usually congenital and is often located around the arch. It may be associated with other congenital abnormalities (e.g. bicuspid aortic valve or PDA). During the examination, check for radio-femoral delay and all peripheral pulses. You would expect reduced pulsation and blood pressure distal to the coarctation.

Cushing's disease (Cushing's syndrome)

Cushing's syndrome refers to elevated circulating cortisol levels of any cause. Cushing's disease specifically refers to a pituitary adenoma causing ACTH and subsequently cortisol release (in 70% of cases). Both present with signs and symptoms of cortisol excess (central obesity, easy bruising, striae, hirsutism, psychiatric disturbance, insulin resistance, etc.). Don't forget to enquire about exogenous steroid use.

Conn's syndrome

Primary hyperaldosteronism may be due to adrenal hyperplasia (this is common), adrenal carcinoma or a benign adenoma. Conn's syndrome specifically refers to the latter. Suspect this if there is a finding of high sodium and low potassium levels without another cause.

Renal artery stenosis

This may be congenital or acquired, unilateral or bilateral, and focal or diffuse. The commonest cause is atherosclerosis, presenting in middle age. Often hypertension worsens and is refractory to medical treatment, and renal function can acutely deteriorate with ACE inhibitors. Renal artery stenosis may be associated with renal bruit.

Cerebrovascular malformation

Rarely a cerebrovascular malformation can cause hypertension via local pressure effects.

Carcinoid syndrome

This is associated with approximately 10% of neuroendocrine tumours.

Patients often have symptoms of flushing, abdominal pain and diarrhoea. In the heart there may be tricuspid and pulmonary regurgitation as the leaflets become restricted.

Clinical examination

Clinical examination of patients with hypertension should include the following:

- Eyes – to look for hypertensive changes in the retina (*see* Table 14.1).
- Abdomen – listen for renal bruits, and palpate for masses.
- Vascular – radio-radio or radio-femoral delay in coarctation.
- Respiratory and cardiovascular – look for evidence of heart failure (this is especially important in patients with acute hypertensive crisis).

TABLE 14.1 Grades of hypertensive retinopathy

Grade I	Silver wiring
Grade II	Grade I + AV nipping
Grade III	Grade II + cotton wool spots and flame haemorrhages
Grade IV	Grade III + papilloedema

Initial investigations

Initial tests for hypertension should look for evidence of end-organ damage and assess cardiovascular risk. Evidence of end-organ damage is particularly important in hypertensive crises.

- **Non-invasive blood pressure.** Refer to the NICE guidelines for the current classification of hypertension. Ensure that measurements are accurate and reproducible. Recent exercise, caffeine intake, smoking or stress can influence readings. Cuff size is important. It should cover two-thirds of the upper arm and the bladder should encircle three-quarters of the circumference. If the cuff is too small, blood pressure can be overestimated. Bilateral readings should be taken if the measurements are high.
- **FBC.** Anaemia is a sign of chronic renal failure.
- **U&E.** Raised creatinine levels indicate end-organ damage. Low potassium levels are found in Conn's syndrome.
- **TFT.** Hyperthyroidism can result in hypertension.
- **Urine.** Proteinuria with or without haematuria is indicative of end-organ damage and renovascular HTN. High urinary potassium levels indicate aldosterone excess.

- **ECG.** Look for left ventricular hypertrophy/strain, and atrial fibrillation.
- **Chest X-ray.** Look for coarctation (rib notching), dissection (widened mediastinum) and cardiac size.
- **Echocardiogram.** Aortic root enlargement (with or without aortic regurgitation), left ventricular hypertrophy, and systolic and/or diastolic dysfunction. Estimate the pulmonary pressure.

Further investigations

If secondary causes of hypertension are suspected, further tests may be required.

- **Plasma renin.** Elevated levels are found in 75% of patients with renovascular disease. This must be done with the patient lying down, and the sample should be taken to the lab immediately on ice.
- **Aldosterone level.** The ratio of plasma aldosterone to renin activity is raised in primary hyperaldosteronism.
- **Cortisol.** Raised serum cortisol levels are found in Cushing's syndrome. This alone is not diagnostic, but it may help to confirm suspicions. Remember that you can't measure a cortisol level if the patient is on exogenous corticosteroids!
- **Dexamethasone suppression test.** Patients with Cushing's syndrome cannot suppress their cortisol levels in response to a dexamethasone suppression test.
- **Urinary catecholamines.** Phaeochromocytoma results in raised levels of urinary catecholamines. Discuss this with the biochemistry laboratory before sending them urine to be tested, as specific bottles are required.
- **Urinary 5-HIAA.** Elevated 24-hour urine levels of 5-HIAA (5-hydroxyindoleacetic acid (5-HIAA) suggest carcinoid. Discuss this with the biochemistry laboratory before sending them urine to be tested, as specific bottles are required.
- **Renal ultrasound.** Kidney size, and Doppler assessment to detect RAS, but it is not as sensitive as MRA (see below). Can be difficult in obese patients.
- **Magnetic resonance angiography (MRA).** This is more sensitive and specific than renal USS for detection of RAS.
- **Ambulatory blood pressure monitoring.** This is useful in cases of white-coat hypertension, and also to monitor the effectiveness of

antihypertensive treatment over a 24-hour period in more difficult hypertensive patients.

Diagnostic criteria

We recommend that you refer to the latest NICE guidelines or the British Hypertension Society guidelines (which are slightly different). Broadly speaking, the most important NICE criteria to remember are as follows:
- Target 140/90 mmHg, *or* 140/80 mmHg if the patient is diabetic.

Management

Medical management

Lifestyle measures

Advise the patient to lose weight, stop smoking, take regular exercise, adopt a healthy diet, and reduce their salt and alcohol intake.

Pharmacological agents

Drugs are indicated if the patient's blood pressure is:
- more than 160/100 mmHg, *or*
- more than 140/90 mmHg and there is end-organ damage or the 10-year cardiovascular (CV) risk is 20%, *or*
- more than 140/80 mmHg if the patient is diabetic with end-organ damage or a 10-year CV risk of 15%.

It is advisable to prescribe once-daily formulations if possible, to try to maximise compliance, especially as 50% of patients will need more than one drug to achieve the target blood pressure.

First-line treatment

- Patients aged < 55 years: ACE inhibitor (or A2RB if intolerant). Beta-blockers are used if there is a contraindication to the use of ACEi and A2RB (e.g. pregnancy).
- Patients aged > 55years: thiazide diuretic or calcium-channel blocker.

Note: Black (African or Caribbean origin) patients should be included in the second group regardless of age.

Second-line treatment

- ACEi + calcium-channel blocker *or* ACEi + diuretic

Third-line treatment

* Add whichever drug has not been used so far (ACEi, calcium-channel blocker or diuretic).

Fourth-line treatment

* Adding a fourth agent would usually involve specialist input. Spironolactone, alpha-blockers and beta-blockers can be considered.

TABLE 14.2 Drug classes and dosing ranges

Class	Drug	Starting dose	Maximum dose
ACE inhibitors	Ramipril	1.25 mg once daily	10 mg/day
	Lisinopril	5 mg once daily	40 mg/day
	Captopril	25 mg once daily	150 mg/day
	Enalapril	5 mg once daily	40 mg/day
Angiotensin-2-receptor blockers	Losartan	25 mg once daily	100 mg/day
	Valsartan	40 mg once daily	160 mg/day
	Candesartan	4 mg once daily	16 mg/day
Diuretics	Bendrofluazide	2.5 mg once daily	5 mg/day
Calcium-channel blockers	Amlodipine	5 mg once daily	10 mg/day
	Diltiazem	60 mg once daily	240 mg/day
	Nifedipine	10 mg three times a day	60 mg/day
Beta-blockers	Atenolol	25 mg once daily	100 mg/day
	Bisoprolol	1.25 mg once daily	10 mg/day

New drugs

* Aliskiren – direct renin inhibitor.
* Eplerenone – aldosterone blocker.
* Bosentan – endothelin-receptor blocker.

Other drugs

* Statins – there is evidence for treating raised lipids in the context of hypertension to reduce the overall cardiovascular risk. The aim is to lower total cholesterol levels by 25% or LDL-cholesterol levels by 30%, or to reach a total cholesterol level of < 4.0 mmol/l or an LDL-cholesterol level of < 2.0 mmol/l.

- Aspirin – HTN is associated with platelet activation and endothelial dysfunction, resulting in a prothrombotic state. Aspirin should be prescribed if there is end-organ damage, diabetes, or the 10-year CV risk is > 20%.

Surgical management
Renal artery stenosis
This may be managed percutaneously or by open surgery. Angioplasty is the first choice, but patients with diffuse disease may do better with surgery.

Primary hyperaldosteronism
Surgical resection (adrenalectomy) is the first-choice procedure. Alternatively, an aldosterone blocker (spironolactone) may be used.

Phaeochromocytoma
Patients are stabilised initially on an alpha-blocker, followed by beta-blocker therapy. Surgical resection is then performed.

Special scenarios
Malignant hypertension
Accelerated or severe hypertension > 220/120 mmHg requires urgent treatment and often hospital admission, especially if cardiac complications (e.g. MI, heart failure) or neurological complications (e.g. haemorrhage, encephalopathy, visual loss) are present. Admit the patient with IV access and cardiac monitoring, often to an HDU setting. Aim to reduce the blood pressure by 25% over a period of 24–48 hours. Intravenous vasodilators (e.g. sodium nitroprusside) or beta-blockers (e.g. labetalol) are usually the first-line treatment, with the addition of calcium-channel blockers or ACE inhibitors systemically.

Hypertension in pregnancy
This may be pre-existing or related to the pregnancy itself. It is the commonest medical problem during pregnancy, and a major cause of maternal mortality. Commonly used drugs include methyldopa, labetalol, nifedipine, clonidine, diuretics and hydralazine. Magnesium is used in the management of pre-eclampsia. Specialist care shared between the cardiologist and obstetricians is often required.

Information to have to hand for ward rounds

Patients are rarely admitted because of hypertension alone. They are only likely to be inpatients if they have been admitted for investigation of secondary causes (although much of this is usually undertaken in outpatient departments), or in the event of hypertensive crisis.

If you have a new patient with hypertension, it is important to be familiar with the following:
- aetiology
- investigations
- treatment to date (including unsuccessful and/or untolerated therapy)
- evidence of end-organ damage.

Too often hypertension is overlooked, but good diagnosis and management will save lives, and impress your consultant.

Further reading

- National Institute for Health and Clinical Excellence. *Hypertension: management of hypertension in adults in primary care.* NICE Clinical Guideline 34. London: NICE; 2006.
- Williams B, Poulter NR, Brown MJ *et al.* British Hypertension Society guidelines for hypertension management 2004 (BHS-IV): summary. *BMJ.* 2004; **328:** 634–40.

15

Aortic syndromes

Aetiology
A number of different pathologies can result in aortic disease:
- inherited (Marfan's syndrome, Ehlers–Danlos syndrome)
- degenerative
- atherosclerotic
- inflammatory
- traumatic.

Whatever the pathology, these mechanisms weaken the arterial wall and result in increased wall stress and aortic dilatation. There is a spectrum of disease that ultimately ends in aortic rupture. Prevention of disease progression is important, as is the management of acute dissection or rupture.

Clinical presentation
Symptoms usually indicate advanced-stage disease (i.e. impending rupture). Otherwise the diagnosis is often incidental, made during imaging investigations (e.g. chest X-ray, echo, CT) that are often being performed for another reason. The aorta is measured at standard places (*see* Figure 15.1). You will see these on the report:
1 AV annulus
2 sinus of Valsalva
3 sinotubular junction
4 ascending aorta.

Normal values depend on which imaging modality is used.

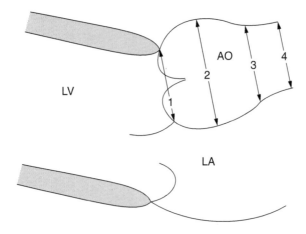

FIGURE 15.1 Measurements of the aorta.

Warning symptoms of acute dissection include the following:
- abrupt-onset chest pain, typically most severe at the time of onset
- pain can be retrosternal (type A) or radiate to the back (type B)
- a sensation of tearing or stabbing
- hypertension
- late presentation can be with heart failure (severe aortic regurgitation), syncope (tamponade) or neurological sequelae.

Signs of acute dissection depend on anatomical location and extent, and include the following:
- unequal blood pressure and pulse volume in the upper limbs
- acute renal failure (if it extends to the renal arteries)
- acute MI (if it extends to the coronary arteries)
- acute aortic regurgitation (if it extends to the aortic root)
- acute stroke (if it extends to the carotid arteries).

The diagnosis can be made at any stage of disease. Screening for pre-clinical disease is performed in patients at risk of developing aortic disease. Table 15.1 shows the features associated with the various aortic syndromes.

TABLE 15.1 Features associated with the different aortic syndromes

Marfan's syndrome	May be detected by family screening. Other features: tall, slender limbs, long digits, chest wall deformity, eye problems, high arched palate
Ehlers–Danlos syndrome	Other features: joint hypermobility, tissue fragility, skin laxity
Atherosclerotic	Hypertension is the main risk factor. Smoking and hypercholesterolaemia are also important
Inflammatory	Large- and medium-vessel vasculitis can affect the aorta (Behçet's disease, Takayasu's arteritis, giant-cell arteritis, rheumatoid arthritis). Syphilis. Cocaine and amphetamine use
Trauma	Usually high-speed deceleration injuries. Also consider after blunt chest trauma or CPR

Initial investigations

Don't delay! The most appropriate investigation will depend on how sick the patient is.

- **FBC.** This may be entirely normal, or reveal anaemia in the context of an underlying chronic inflammatory process. A reactive thrombocytosis may be present.
- **U&E.** Renal function may be abnormal if there is an extensive vasculitis involving the kidneys.
- **Clotting screen.** The patient may require surgery.
- **Group and save.** Aortic bleeds can be catastrophic within minutes. Patients should have a routine group and save as a minimum. In the event of surgery, liaise with the surgeons about the number of units they would like cross-matched.
- **Autoimmune screen.** ANCA, ANA, ENA, rheumatoid factor and ESR should be sent early. The results of these tests often take some time to come back.
- **Syphilis screen.** VDRL, rapid plasma regain (RPR) and TPHA.
- **ECG.** Look for evidence of ischaemia. Inferior ischaemic changes are the typical finding with dissection.
- **Chest X-ray.** Look for evidence of a widened mediastinum. This is not enough to confirm or exclude your diagnosis, but it may help.

Further investigations

Further imaging depends on local availability and expertise. The goal is to confirm the diagnosis, classify the dissection, identify the true and false lumen, and detect side branch involvement. Options for further investigative imaging include the following:

- echocardiography
- CT
- MRI.

In cases of haemodynamic instability, the patient requires intubation, urgent surgical consultation and a TOE.

Diagnostic criteria

There are various classification systems that you may see in reports.
The Stanford classification describes location:

- type A – involves the ascending aorta, and requires urgent surgical management
- type B – involves the descending aorta, and can be managed medically.

The DeBakey classification describes extent:

- type I – involves the entire aorta
- type II – involves the ascending aorta
- type III – involves the descending aorta.

There are also different subtypes, depending on the pathogenesis:

- class I – classic dissection with intimal flap between true and false lumen
- class II – disruption of the media with intramural haematoma
- class III – discrete dissection without haematoma, and only a bulge is seen
- class IV – plaque rupture and aortic ulceration
- class V – traumatic or iatrogenic.

Management

Medical management

As with any potentially sick patient, this should follow the initial ABC approach. Thereafter, pain relief is extremely important. Once the diagnosis has been made, the patient must be transferred to the intensive care unit and the cardiothoracic surgeons made aware of this. Patients with type A dissection may go straight to theatre. Those with type B dissection will usually be managed medically.

The next step is to lower the blood pressure in order to reduce wall stress and reduce the risk of rupture. Short-acting beta-blockers (e.g. propranolol, metoprolol, esmolol) are used. Calcium-channel blockers are first-line treatment if beta-blockers are contraindicated. Nitrates or sodium nitroprusside can be added if the patient remains hypertensive. Aim for a systolic blood pressure of 100–120 mmHg. Intra-arterial blood pressure monitoring may be required.

Surgical management

The aim of surgical repair is to prevent aortic rupture, severe aortic regurgitation and pericardial tamponade. Various techniques are performed. A knowledge of the size of the aortic root and the condition of the aortic valve is essential when planning surgery. Modern techniques also include percutaneous stent placement, and are usually performed in tertiary centres as a joint procedure by cardiac and vascular surgeons.

Prevention

The likelihood of aortic dissection can be reduced in those at risk (i.e. patients with Marfan's syndrome, Ehlers–Danlos syndrome or hypertension). Progression from asymptomatic aortic dilatation can be slowed by the following:

- lifelong beta-blockers
- serial aortic imaging
- prophylactic surgery if the aortic root measures > 5.5 cm or 5 cm (if there is a family history)
- moderate restriction of physical activity.

The prognosis for aortic dissection is improving all the time, but is still poor. Around 20% of patients die before reaching hospital. Of those that do reach hospital, 50% die within the first 48 hours. Rapid diagnosis and treatment is the key to improving the prognosis.

Daily monitoring and investigations

1 Close observations of vital signs in an ICU setting.
2 Daily examination, looking specifically for any new cardiac murmurs, peripheral pulses or new neurological signs.
3 Daily ECG, looking for ischaemic changes.
4 Daily bloods, including FBC, U&E and CRP.

Important tips

Surgeons

Discuss cases with the surgeons as soon as the diagnosis is suspected, so that they are aware of the patient. They are likely to want to see the patient even if it is a type B dissection, as the dissection flap may extend back towards the arch.

Information to have to hand for ward rounds

1 Up-to-date bloods, including FBC, U&E, CRP and ESR.
2 Daily ECG, with a knowledge of what it shows.
3 The results of the most recent echocardiogram and any other imaging.
4 Observation chart for temperature and haemodynamic status.

16

Cardiogenic shock

Epidemiology

Cardiogenic shock (CS) is the most common cause of death among inpatients with acute myocardial infarction. Although high, mortality rates are declining, and this is thought to be a result of increasing utilisation of re-perfusion therapy, revascularisation, and haemodynamic support with intra-aortic balloon pumping (IABP).

Aetiology

More often than not, cardiogenic shock is a result of an extensive acute myocardial infarction. Other important causes of cardiogenic shock include the following:

- arrhythmia
- aortic dissection
- acute valvular destruction (e.g. endocarditis)
- myocarditis
- cardiac tamponade
- pulmonary embolism
- tension pneumothorax.

Cardiogenic shock has an extremely poor prognosis, with a high mortality. Therefore diagnosis and prompt management are of utmost importance.

Clinical presentation

Patients may present in a number of different ways, but the ability to recognise the acutely unwell patient is a skill that must be learned quickly and soundly. Assessment should include the following.

General inspection
- Often pale, with the skin having a waxy or mottled appearance.
- Cool peripheries.
- Clammy.

Level of consciousness
- Patients will often have a reduced GCS score.

Pulse
- Tachycardia.
- Assess for rate, rhythm and character.
- Patients may have pulsus alternans (in which arterial pulse waveform shows alternating higher and lower pressures; sign of severe LV systolic dysfunction), pulsus paradoxus (an exaggeration of the normal decrease in systolic blood pressure of > 10 mmHg), or a low-volume pulse.
- Palpate all of the peripheral pulses, as dissection may result in the loss of unilateral peripheral pulses.

Jugular venous pressure
- This may be difficult to assess and/or interpret in CS.
- Generally unhelpful when assessing volume status in patients suffering CS. The change in JVP or CVP measured using a central line in response to fluid challenge is more helpful. If the JVP or CVP is low, but rises with fluid (e.g. 100 ml IV administered over 10 minutes) and then falls again, it is likely that the patient is underfilled. If it rises and remains that way, the patient is likely to be relatively euvolaemic.
- Extreme care should be taken when giving intravenous fluid in these circumstances, and this should only be done under supervision by a senior doctor.
- The JVP is likely to be elevated in patients with pulmonary embolus or right ventricular infarction, and normal in those with anterior myocardial infarct (unless complicated by pulmonary oedema).
- Assessment of the JVP may be of benefit in patients with cardiac tamponade, demonstrating a paradoxical rise on inspiration (Kussmaul's sign). This occurs because as the intrathoracic pressure becomes more negative on inspiration, the pressure created by the pericardial fluid prevents blood from flowing into the right heart in the

normal fashion. Blood is therefore 'pushed' up the SVC instead, where it is seen as Kussmaul's sign.

Apex beat
- May not be palpable in cardiac tamponade.
- Is displaced with tension pneumothorax (the direction will depend on which side the pneumothorax is).
- Hyperdynamic in the context of acute mitral regurgitation.

Heart sounds
- Muffled in cardiac tamponade and occasionally in left-sided tension pneumothorax.
- Pansystolic murmur in acute mitral regurgitation and VSD (the latter may occur acutely due to large anterior MI).
- S_3 gallop rhythm.

Initial investigations

FBC
This should form part of the routine testing of a patient, but is unlikely to be of any specific benefit. The presence of anaemia increases morbidity and mortality. A raised white cell count (neutrophils) is common with myocardial infarction.

D-dimers
If PE is suspected, these are highly likely to be raised in the very sick shocked patient.

U&E
Renal impairment increases morbidity and mortality. It is important to identify whether renal impairment is a new phenomenon, so always call the GP or look for old results. Hyperkalaemia must be treated aggressively as follows:
- Give 10 ml of 10% calcium gluconate or calcium chloride over 10 minutes IV.
- Give 10 units of Actrapid insulin in 50 ml of 50% glucose over 30 minutes IV.
- Re-check serum potassium levels after treatment. Patients should be on a cardiac monitor during treatment, and until their potassium level has normalised.

Group and save
Some patients may require surgery or cardiac intervention, depending on the aetiology of cardiogenic shock. All patients should have a group and save sent, and patients who are likely to require surgery will need cross-matched blood available (ask the surgeon how many units to cross-match).

Cardiac enzymes
These should be measured at baseline and 12 hours. Some institutions will also check enzymes at 6 hours. A negative initial troponin result does not exclude a cardiac event.

Clotting screen
If the patient is to undergo thrombolysis and has a raised INR, this may preclude treatment. Patients on warfarin (e.g. for a previous PE) must have their clotting checked to ensure that their INR is therapeutic. A PE is relatively uncommon when the INR is therapeutic. Patients who are going for surgery need to have their clotting checked and then corrected as appropriate.

Chest X-ray
- **PE.** This may be completely normal, or reveal a small pleural effusion, peripheral wedge-shaped infarct, etc.
- **Tension pneumothorax.** This is a medical emergency that should be clinically detected and treated, rather than delaying for a chest X-ray. However, the latter would show a mediastinal shift away from the side of the pneumothorax, with loss of the lung markings to the chest wall on the same side of the pneumothorax. A small pleural effusion may also be seen.
- **Cardiac tamponade.** This may reveal the classically described 'boot-shaped' heart.

Transthoracic echocardiogram
This should be requested as an urgent investigation by discussing it directly with the on-call cardiology registrar. TTE is discussed in Chapter 7.

ECG
- **PE.** Sinus tachycardia is the most common feature. There may be signs of right heart strain, such as right axis deviation or ST-segment changes in V1 and V2. The classically described $S_IQ_{III}T_{III}$ is uncommon.
- **Cardiac tamponade.** Electrical alternans may rarely be observed.

More commonly, the only feature consists of small voltage complexes throughout all leads.

- **Myocardial infarction.** ST-segment changes and T-wave inversion in vascular territories (*see* Chapter 7).

Further investigations

Echocardiography

- **Pericardial effusion and cardiac tamponade.** Pericardial fluid is usually well detected by echocardiography. Tamponade is a clinical diagnosis, although echocardiography provides supporting evidence such as right atrial and/or right ventricular diastolic collapse. Remember that not all effusions cause tamponade.
- **Aortic syndromes.** Echocardiography is a useful first investigation where promptly available to assess proximal aortic root dimensions, the presence of aortic regurgitation and any associated effusion. The aortic arch can also often be seen.
- **Pulmonary embolism.** A massive PE may cause signs of right-sided pressure overload on echocardiography, including dilated right atrium and right ventricle, tricuspid regurgitation and raised pulmonary pressure. Occasionally embolus may be directly visualised in the right heart. The proximal pulmonary trunk can usually be seen with echocardiography.
- **Myocardial infarction.** Regional wall motion abnormalities may be evident. Inspection of the valvular apparatus is important in the context of acute valvular incompetence. Extensive right ventricular infarcts may result in cardiogenic shock.
- **Critical valvular disease.** Less commonly CS may be the mode of presentation of critical valvular disease (e.g. aortic stenosis).

CTPA

It is generally only massive PEs that result in cardiogenic shock. The investigation of choice in this instance would be CTPA. There is no place for VQ scanning. The patient *must* be stabilised before this investigation is performed! A combination of other investigations such as arterial blood gas, echocardiography, chest X-ray and ECG may be all that is required to thrombolyse the PE, thus rendering the CTPA unnecessary. This is a management decision that can only be made by a senior doctor.

Cardiac rhythm monitoring

Arrhythmias may be detected as the cause of cardiogenic shock, and should be managed in accordance with the current guidelines from the UK Resuscitation Council. All ventricular arrhythmias and accessory pathways, including pre-excited arrhythmia, should be discussed with a cardiologist.

CT aortic angiography

This is a contrast-enhanced CT scan of the aorta which may be used to detect aortic dissection with a high degree of sensitivity and specificity. The patient *must* be stabilised before being sent through a scanner. The anaesthetists should be made aware of the situation in case the patient requires rapid intubation.

Management

Medical management

The management of patients with cardiogenic shock must be rapid. These patients are extremely sick and require a high level of attention. Contact your seniors as soon as you suspect that a patient may have cardiogenic shock, and contact the cardiology specialist registrar on call immediately.

Daily monitoring/investigations

1   Close observations of vital signs and daily weights (routine in ICU or HDU).
2   Daily examination of cardiovascular and respiratory systems.
3   Daily bloods – U&E and magnesium levels should be closely monitored when patients are on high doses of diuretics. This is especially important in patients on furosemide infusions. LFT should be monitored in case ischaemic hepatitis develops secondary to a low cardiac output state.
4   Cardiac output studies – there are numerous different methods of measuring cardiac output, but this subject is well beyond the remit of this book.

Important tips

ICU

These patients are extremely unwell and must be managed in an HDU or ICU setting. To ensure that a patient is appropriately managed, inform the ICU team and ensure that they are aware that the patient is likely to require their input. Speak to them early on!

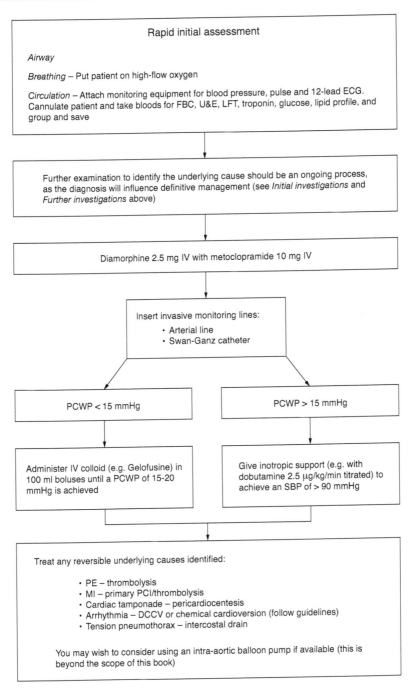

FIGURE 16.1 Management of cardiogenic shock.

Cardiology

Discuss any patients with suspected cardiogenic shock with the cardiology specialist registrar on call, as they will need to do an urgent echocardiogram. Depending upon the cause, the patient may require urgent pericardiocentesis. The cardiologists may also wish to insert an intra-aortic balloon pump.

Information to have to hand for ward rounds

1 Up-to-date bloods, including FBC, U&E, LFT and cardiac enzymes.
2 ECG from the current admission together with any previous ECGs. This is particularly important in cases of cardiogenic shock resulting from ischaemia.
3 The results of the most recent echocardiogram.
4 The results of all previous cardiac investigations.
5 Observation chart for haemodynamic status.

17

Myocardial and pericardial disease

Hypertrophic cardiomyopathy

Aetiology

HCM is the commonest inherited heart disease, affecting 1 in 500 people worldwide. It is caused by mutations encoding sarcomeric proteins, and is inherited in an autosomal dominant pattern. The condition classically presents with symptoms in the late teens or early adulthood, usually exertional breathlessness, syncope or palpitations. However, the diagnosis is often made after the incidental finding of a murmur or abnormal ECG. Increasingly the diagnosis is made through family or pre-participation sports screening.

Diagnosis

The diagnosis is a clinical one, and is based on the finding of unexplained ventricular hypertrophy > 15 mm (or > 13 mm if there is a family history of HCM). It is important to consider and exclude other causes of left ventricular hypertrophy (e.g. hypertension, valve disease, athlete's heart, metabolic disease and amyloid).

ECG

This typically shows prominent voltage in all leads, septal Q-waves and repolarisation abnormalities. Around 5–10% of patients may have a normal-looking ECG.

Echocardiography

There is usually asymmetrical septal hypertrophy, but an apical distribution and concentric hypertrophy are compatible with the diagnosis. Other features to look for are small LV cavity, large left atrium and diastolic dysfunction. Outflow tract obstruction is present at rest in over 50% of cases, but may require stress (valsalva or exercise) to unmask it. Other typical features include SAM (systolic anterior motion of the mitral valve) and posteriorly directed mitral regurgitation.

Management
There are four important aspects of management:
1 **Prevention of sudden cardiac death.** This is based on risk stratification. The presence of two or more risk factors (LVH > 3 cm, LVOTO, syncope, abnormal exercise blood pressure response, NSVT or family history of sudden cardiac death) is associated with an annual mortality of 5%, and an ICD is indicated.
2 **Relief of symptoms.** Negatively inotropic drugs such as beta-blockers and calcium-channel blockers are the first-line treatment. Disopyramide can be used in addition.
3 **Relief of outflow tract obstruction.** Strategies for doing this include DDD pacing, alcohol septal ablation and surgical myectomy.
4 **Family screening.** All first-degree relatives should be offered screening with ECG and echocardiography. Lifelong follow-up is recommended, with screening every 5 years in adulthood, as late-onset disease within families is recognised.

Prognosis
For the majority of patients the prognosis is good, with normal life expectancy. However, a small percentage of patients develop progressive heart failure and dilatation. Their prognosis is worse, and cardiac transplantation may be needed.

Dilated cardiomyopathy
Aetiology
This is the commonest cardiomyopathy, and it can be the consequence of hypertensive, ischaemic, valvular or congenital heart disease. Other causes include the following:
- drugs (anthracyclines, alcohol and cocaine)
- myocarditis (viral and autoimmune)
- peripartum (defined as between 1 month before and 5 months after delivery)

- inherited/familial
- sarcoid
- metabolic (haemochromatosis, hyperthyroid, thiamine deficiency, sepsis)
- arrhythmias (atrial fibrillation, frequent ectopy)
- iron overload (recurrent transfusions in sickle and thalassaemia patients).

Diagnosis

Based on echocardiography, LV cavity size should be indexed to body surface area. The diagnosis depends on EF < 45% and LVEDD > 117% predicted for body size. Ejection fraction is more closely linked to prognosis than overall cardiac size.

TABLE 17.1 Investigations used for diagnostic and prognostic assessment

Laboratory tests	FBC, U&Es, LFT, GGT, TFTs, CK, serum ACE, ferritin, ESR, CRP, ANA and viral screen (coxsackie, EBV and HIV)
Echocardiogram	Chamber size, ejection fraction, wall thickness, valve disease and regional wall motion abnormalities
ECG	Previous infarct, complex size, conduction disease and arrhythmias
Holter monitor	Ectopic burden, paroxysmal arrhythmias or conduction disease
Cardiac MRI	Can detect fibrosis and scarring. Specific patterns are associated with infarction, sarcoid and myocarditis
Coronary angiogram	To exclude ischaemic heart disease
TOE	Helpful for assessing complex valve pathology or looking for thrombus
Stress echo	To assess contractile reserve, which correlates with prognosis
Endomyocardial biopsy	May be helpful in diagnosis, but yield is low and rarely changes management

Management

This is similar to the standard treatment for heart failure. There is evidence that ACE inhibitors and beta-blockers improve survival. Spironolactone should be added if NYHA class III or IV. Diuretic therapy may be needed for symptomatic benefit. Specific treatments may be added in certain situation (e.g. chelation for iron overload, steroids for sarcoidosis). Device therapy (CRT and or ICD) should be considered in those who meet conventional criteria. Current NICE guidelines recommend that CRT should be considered if the following criteria are met:

- NYHA class III or IV
- LVEF ≤ 35%
- QRS > 120 ms
- patient is on optimal medical therapy.

Prognosis

This is related to the severity of disease at presentation and the underlying aetiology. Renal impairment, EF < 35%, broad QRS, anaemia and reduced exercise capacity confer a worse prognosis.

Restrictive cardiomyopathy

This is the least common cardiomyopathy. It is characterised by a stiff heart muscle with reduced LV cavity size, which requires a high filling pressure to maintain cardiac output. Restrictive ventricular physiology also occurs in other cardiomyopathies. The commonest cause in the western world is amyloid, and in the tropics it is endomyocardial fibrosis. Other infiltrative causes include haemochromatosis, sarcoid and glycogen storage diseases. There is no evidence that standard heart failure therapy (ACE inhibitors and beta-blockers) improves the prognosis, and treatment is often targeted at symptom relief with diuretics. The condition is usually progressive, and has a poor prognosis.

Arrhythmogenic right ventricular cardiomyopathy

Arrhythmogenic right ventricular cardiomyopathy (ARVC) is an inherited heart muscle disease characterised by myocyte loss with fatty or fibro-fatty replacement. It can affect both the left and right ventricle, and is caused by mutations in desmosomal proteins. It is associated with ventricular arrhythmias, congestive heart failure and sudden cardiac death. Diagnosis is based on a number of major and minor criteria. T-wave inversion in the right precordial leads V2 and V3 should make you suspect the diagnosis. A patient with known ARVC presenting with increasing symptoms of arrhythmias should usually be admitted for cardiac monitoring and a specialist opinion. Anti-arrhythmic medication and ICD are used to reduce the risk of ventricular arrhythmia.

Pericarditis

This typically presents with chest pain (classically sharp, pleuritic, and relieved by sitting forward) and sometimes fever. There may be a history of a viral illness, recent MI or new drugs. On examination look for signs of haemodynamic compromise and underlying aetiology.

Investigations

These are directed at excluding important underlying diagnoses (e.g. malignancy, infection, autoimmune disease).

- Laboratory tests should include FBC, LFT, CRP, ESR, and thyroid, autoimmune and viral screen.
- ECG may mimic a myocardial infarction with ST elevation. Specific features that are more supportive of pericarditis are PR depression and global changes (*see* Figure 17.1).
- Chest X-ray to look for lung masses or aortic aneurysm.
- An echocardiogram to confirm the presence or absence of a pericardial effusion.

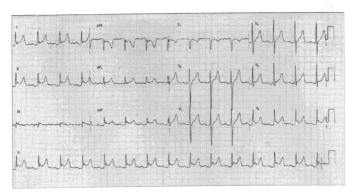

FIGURE 17.1 ECG showing typical saddle-shaped ST segments in pericarditis.

Management

This is usually a self-limiting illness, and it can be treated with anti-inflammatory medication (NSAIDs, high-dose aspirin or colchicine). Drainage may be required for diagnostic purposes or if there is haemodynamic compromise. This can often be done percutaneously, but if the effusion is malignant (and therefore likely to recur), localised or the patient is significantly obese, it may be best done surgically, with the creation of a pericardial window.

Prognosis

This is usually good and no long-term follow-up is required. If recurrent, a constrictive pericarditis may develop.

Cardiac tamponade

This is a clinical diagnosis and it requires urgent treatment. Beck's triad of muffled heart sounds, hypotension and raised JVP is typical. Other signs include pulsus paradoxus, low-voltage ECG and shock. Urgent drainage is required. Fluids should be given while waiting for the procedure to optimise LV filling.

Index

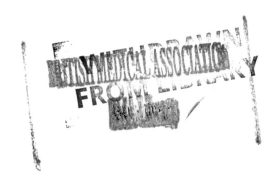